healthy, happy
*pregnancy*
cookbook

# healthy, happy *pregnancy* cookbook

over 125 delicious recipes to satisfy you, nourish baby,
and combat common pregnancy discomforts

### stephanie clarke, RD and willow jarosh, RD

**ATRIA** PAPERBACK

NEW YORK   LONDON   TORONTO   SYDNEY   NEW DELHI

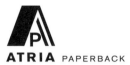

**ATRIA** PAPERBACK

An Imprint of Simon & Schuster, Inc.
1230 Avenue of the Americas
New York, NY 10020

First Atria Paperback edition September 2016

ATRIA PAPERBACK and colophon are trademarks of Simon & Schuster, Inc.

For information about special discounts for bulk purchases, please contact Simon & Schuster Special Sales at 1-866-506-1949 or business@simonandschuster.com.

The Simon & Schuster Speakers Bureau can bring authors to your live event. For more information or to book an event contact the Simon & Schuster Speakers Bureau at 1-866-248-3049 or visit our website at www.simonspeakers.com.

Interior design by Amy Trombat

Manufactured in the United States of America

10 9 8 7 6 5 4 3 2

Library of Congress Cataloging-in-Publication Data
Names: Clarke, Stephanie, author. | Jarosh, Willow, author.
Title: Healthy, happy pregnancy cookbook : over 125 delicious recipes to satisfy you, nourish baby, and combat common pregnancy discomforts / Stephanie Clarke, MS, RD & Willow Jarosh, MS, RD.
Description: First Atria paperback edition. | New York : Atria Books, 2016.
Identifiers: LCCN 2016015142 (print) | LCCN 2016015982 (ebook) |
Subjects: LCSH: Pregnancy—Nutritional aspects. | Mothers—Nutrition. |
BISAC: HEALTH & FITNESS / Pregnancy & Childbirth. | COOKING / Specific Ingredients / Natural Foods. | HEALTH & FITNESS / Nutrition. | LCGFT: Cookbooks.
Classification: LCC RG559. C55 2016 (print) | LCC RG559 (ebook) | DDC 618.²/₄₂—dc23
LC record available at https://lccn.loc.gov/2016015142

ISBN 978-1-5011-3091-5

ISBN 978-1-5011-3093-9 (ebook)

To all moms-to-be and the people who love them.
A great adventure awaits.

# Contents

# healthy, happy
## *pregnancy*
### cookbook

# Introduction

Major congratulations are in order! You've just scored an amazing new gig as the CEO of a new start-up. This will likely be in addition to one or more existing jobs—let the multitasking begin! Your new assignment involves your body taking on the exciting forty-week challenge of growing the next generation of (insert your last name here). Whether it's your first or fifth baby, this will without a doubt be an experience like no other. And while there will be many magical moments, like any job worth having, there will be aspects that will come in the form of some not-so-magical side effects. We're talking about nausea, "cankles," and constipation, to name a few. All the while you'll be tasked with something very important—eating right to nourish you and your baby in the best way possible.

On that note, we introduce you to the *Healthy, Happy Pregnancy Cookbook*, organized by common pregnancy symptoms. Like any other cookbook, these chapters are filled with recipes—delicious recipes. But unlike any other cookbook, these recipes all contain ingredients that deliver the nutrients your body needs to combat the most common pregnancy discomforts while nourishing baby in the healthiest way possible. It's an "eat-to-beat" way of looking at your meals and snacks. As a crazy-powerful (or is that crazy, powerful?) CEO, these nutrients are your employees. And while the tone of this book doesn't take itself too seriously, we take your needs very seriously. So you can laugh while you whip up truly healing meals.

These recipes are free of overly processed ingredients and filled with whole foods. This means that when eating these meals you'll be avoiding an excess of processed carbs, too much added sugar and sodium, and fewer icky additives, all of which can impact your (and your baby's) health, as well as how you feel in the short and long term. Clean eating is a term that is thrown around all the time but has, until this cookbook, never been applied to pregnancy. And you don't have to special-order obscure, ridiculously expensive ingredients to make these meals. We had you in mind when we created them and we respect your time and your bank account while also believing that you deserve the most delicious, nutritious, healing food. Think of these recipes as a reflection of you—they multitask, they get a whole lot accomplished, and they have great taste.

Last but not least, these recipes can be used for years and years after your pregnancy, so we hope they become favorites for your entire family. Someday that little poppy seed-, or kiwi-, or cantaloupe-size human inside of you might just make you Mother's Day breakfast from this book.

Be healthy. Be happy.


Written with love,
Stephanie Clarke, MS, RD and Willow Jarosh, MS, RD

# Basics

## Nutrition Dos and Don'ts During Pregnancy

### DO commit to adopting these healthy habits

Pregnancy is the perfect time to say sayonara to not-so-stellar eating habits. Focus on these, and you'll be feeding you and baby right.

1. **Don't skip:** Eat consistent meals throughout the day. Don't skip meals or wait more than 4 to 5 hours without eating anything. This will also help keep your energy levels more consistently high, and keep nausea at bay.

2. **Rise and dine:** Eat breakfast. Baby is growing around the clock, so skipping breakfast means baby is missing important growing materials. Having a hard time with nausea? Visit chapter 1 for recipes to help you squeeze in some nutrition when all you feel like eating are saltines. In general, try a cold fruit smoothie like the Peach-Ginger Smoothie (page 45), or anything that doesn't make your stomach cringe. It doesn't have to be traditional breakfast food.

3. **Stay well hydrated:** This is one of the things that will make a huge difference in how you feel during pregnancy. Daily adequate water intake is important for vital body functions such as digestion, circulation, regularity, nutrient absorption, and much more. Water is essential to help transport nutrients through your blood to your baby. Proper hydration can prevent pregnancy-related symptoms such as constipation and hemorrhoids, excessive leg swelling caused by water retention, leg cramps, and dry skin. How much water do you need? Start with at least 8 cups per day (64 ounces) and add an additional 1 cup of water for every 1 hour of light activity. Then give yourself the urine-color test. If your urine is light to clear, you're doing well staying hydrated. If it's a dark yellow to brown (like apple juice) you need to drink more water.

Healthy, Happy Pregnancy Cookbook

4. Cook more at home: Making more of your meals at home means that you can control what goes into your diet (thankfully, you've got your hands on this cookbook!) and your baby's. Restaurant meals are notoriously high in sodium, which can increase water retention and puffiness. Plus, you'll likely eat a meal that's more calorie-appropriate at home, which will help you maintain a healthy rate of weight gain.

5. Eat mostly nutrient-rich foods: You've got 9-ish months to give baby the best nourishment possible, and because your calorie needs don't actually increase that much (the approximately 400 additional calories a day you need in the second and third trimesters is not all that much food), you should choose those extras wisely. Go for whole foods that are rich in nutrients as opposed to foods that contain empty calories like soda, sweetened beverages, processed grains, and processed baked goods.

## DON'T double your food intake

But how much more should you eat? While you are eating for two during pregnancy, one of those two ranges in size from a poppy seed to a watermelon. (Ouch, don't think about that right now.) So, your calories don't need to be doubled, but they do need to be maximized. In other words, the extra 340 calories a day you need during the second and 450 a day in the third trimesters shouldn't be coming from ice cream and pickles on a regular basis (although there's certainly a place for both of those foods in your diet!). These recipes maximize nutrients so the additional calories you need go toward meeting increased requirements for nutrients like iron, protein, and choline. For more on those VIP nutrients, see page 12.

## DO monitor your weight gain

Gaining weight at an appropriate rate is a good sign that you're doing well in terms of managing your increased hunger with your calorie needs. Your doctor should let you know if you're off track in either direction, however it's important to ask questions about how you're doing at each visit. If you think you're gaining too quickly or not quickly enough, bring it up with your doctor if he or she hasn't already. If you're overweight at the beginning of your pregnancy, speak to your doctor about the recommendations for weight gain and see the chart for weight gain recommendations below. Pregnancy is not a time to cut calories drastically, but you will likely be recommended to gain less weight overall.

# what's my healthy pregnancy weight gain?

**Step 1:** Calculate your pre-pregnancy Body Mass Index (BMI)

How to do this:

1. Multiply your weight in pounds x 703 =
2. Square your height in inches (i.e. height x height) =
3. Then divide step 1 by step 2: weight (pounds) x 703 / height =

For example, a woman who weighs 140 pounds and is 5'5" would have the following BMI calculation:

1. 140 pounds x 703 = 98,420
2. 65 inches x 65 inches = 4225
3. 98,420 / 4225 = 23.29

**Step 2:** Find your BMI on the Chart below to determine your weight gain

| PRE-PREGNANCY BMI | TOTAL WEIGHT GAIN | WEIGHT GAIN 1ST TRIMESTER | WEIGHT GAIN PER WEEK IN 2ND AND 3RD TRIMESTERS |
|---|---|---|---|
| < 18.5 | 28–40 pounds | 5 pounds | ~ 1.2 pounds |
| 18.5–24.9 | 25–35 pounds | 1–5 pounds | ~ 1 pound |
| > 25.0–29.9 | 15–25 pounds | 0–2 pounds | ~ .6 pounds |
| > 30.0 | 11–20 pounds | 0–2 pounds | ~ .6 pounds |
| Twin pregnancy | 34–45 pounds | | ~ 1.5 pounds |
| Triplet pregnancy | 45–55 pounds | | ~ 1.5–2 pounds |

## DON'T consume these foods and drinks

A lot of people think that once you are pregnant there is an endless list of DON'Ts. While it's true that there are a few foods and behaviors that are not recommended, there are so many that are that we highly suggest focusing on all of the healthful foods you CAN eat (starting with the yummy recipes in this book). With that in mind, here's a list of foods and beverages that you should avoid or use caution with.

- Alcohol: Whether to completely abstain from alcohol or if it's safe to have an occasional drink has been recently (and hotly) debated. The majority of health professionals and large health organizations continue to recommend abstinence during pregnancy. It is well documented that drinking in excess is harmful to a growing baby. However, the lines are blurred when it comes to moderate drinking and no set amount has been proven safe. Please discuss this issue with your doctor if you are considering an occasional glass of vino or any other type of alcoholic beverage.

- Too much caffeine: If you're a coffee drinker, you can breathe a sigh of relief because according to current recommendations, you don't have to give up your daily cup of Joe (or opt for a decaf version) entirely. While observational studies have linked excessive caffeine intake to increased risk of miscarriage, large studies do not show a benefit of avoiding caffeine altogether. Most health professionals agree with the March of Dimes recommendations that consuming no more than 200 mg/day is safe for baby. Do keep in mind that coffee shops often serve up larger portions than 8 ounces (a medium coffee at a coffee shop is typically 16 ounces, or 2 cups). And some have higher caffeine levels per cup, such as Starbucks, which has approximately 1.5 times the caffeine content of your typical home brew. We recommend sticking with a "short" cup (8 ounces) of Starbucks. Here is a list of common sources of caffeine and their amounts:

Starbucks Grande Coffee (16 oz) 330 mg

Starbucks Tall Coffee (12 oz) 260 mg

Maxwell House ground coffee brewed (12 oz) 100–160 mg

Dunkin' Donuts Coffee (14 oz/medium) 178 mg

Dr Pepper (12 oz) 37 mg

7-Eleven Big Gulp Diet Coke (32 oz) 124 mg

7-Eleven Big Gulp Coca-Cola (32 oz) 92 mg

Ben & Jerry's Coffee Buzz Ice Cream (8 oz) 72 mg

Baker's chocolate (1 oz) 26 mg

Green tea (6 oz) 40 mg

Black tea (6 oz) 45 mg

Excedrin (per tablet) 65 mg

Source: CSPInet.org and Starbucks.com

Raw fish: We know this is a tough one if you're a sushi lover, so you may be happy to hear that not ALL sushi is off limits. Feel free to enjoy any cooked sushi rolls (many rolls contain cooked shrimp, cooked or raw vegetables, and other types of cooked fish, which we highly encourage—after all, seafood is an important part of a healthy pregnancy) and all of the other healthful options at sushi restaurants (edamame, seaweed salad, miso soup, etc.). When in doubt be sure to ask your server if the fish is raw or cooked in a particular dish. Additionally, while major organizations like the American Congress of Obstetricians and Gynecologists (ACOG) still recommend avoiding raw fish, some experts and doctors are giving their patients leeway as long as the fish has been frozen prior to being served, which is said to reduce the risk of parasites. That said, there's still a risk of getting sick from cross contamination with other bacteria or food-borne pathogens after the fish has been frozen, which means the fish came in contact with another food that was infected. If you want to avoid as much risk as possible, we say skip the raw stuff until after delivery. But this, like all other safety issues during pregnancy, is something you should discuss with your doctor first.

◁ Four types of high-mercury fish: shark, swordfish, tilefish, king mackerel. See sidebar (page 8) for more on seafood recommendations during pregnancy.

◁ Lunch meats and refrigerated smoked fish or pâtés: Refrigerated lunch meat can harbor a bacterium called *Listeria monocytogenes*, which can lead to an infection that can be harmful to baby but may not cause any symptoms in you. While *Listeria* is relatively rare, you're more susceptible to it when you're pregnant. If you're wondering what the heck you're going to eat now that lunch meat is off the table, don't fret. You can still enjoy all of the above as long as they're used in a cooked dish (i.e., casserole, frittata, etc.) or heated until steaming first. That said, it's safer to skip take-out deli meat sandwiches and stick to making them yourself at home—this way you can be sure they were heated properly.

◁ Unpasteurized cheese or any other unpasteurized food: It used to be that pregnant women were told to avoid soft cheeses altogether. But the good news is that you can eat all of the feta, blue cheese, and Brie you want as long as you check the ingredients to confirm that it's been made with pasteurized milk. Or, if you're at a restaurant, ask your server to confirm that it's pasteurized cheese. Other foods and beverages that may not be pasteurized and should be skipped during pregnancy · are bottled unpasteurized apple cider, unpasteurized fruit/veggie juices, and homemade soft cheeses like queso blanco made with unpasteurized milk.

It probably goes without saying, but all of the foods used in this book are safe to eat for women with a normal, healthy pregnancy. Even women with certain conditions such as gestational diabetes will benefit from following these recipes, which provide low amounts of refined carbohydrates and a balance of protein, fat, and high-fiber carbohydrates to help keep your blood sugar as steady as possible. Please, please, please talk with your doctor and/or a registered dietitian about starting any new eating plan if you have gestational diabetes or any other more complicated condition during pregnancy.

# eat more from the sea!

There's a lot of confusing information out there about eating seafood while you're pregnant and nursing—the last thing you need is something else to worry about or avoid. The good news is that you absolutely should not be avoiding seafood. Most seafood is not only safe to eat while pregnant, but also provides crucial nutrients and brain benefits.

Fish is a great source of lean protein and iron, two nutrients particularly important during pregnancy. It's also rich in many other vitamins and minerals including vitamins A and D, selenium, choline, and iodine. What sets fish apart even further, making it so important during pregnancy and lactation, is that it's the predominant dietary source of omega-3 fatty acids, specifically the omega-3 called DHA, which is an essential nutrient in the development of baby's brain and nervous system.

You'll need 200 mg/day of DHA to cover both your needs and baby's. You don't need to get exactly 200 mg in each day, but can average 200 mg/day for the week (i.e., around 1400 mg/week). You can get that in 2 to 3 servings of fatty fish per week. Some of the best sources of omega-3 DHA include fatty fish such as salmon, tuna, sardines, herring, anchovies, and bluefish. Almost all fish contain some DHA, so no matter which ones you enjoy, you're getting a benefit. Eating a variety of seafood, and making sure to include fatty fish, will ensure that you're getting enough omega-3 fats.

So what about mercury and other contaminants? Methylmercury is a toxic metal found in minute amounts in almost all species of fish. In high amounts, this type of mercury can accumulate in mom. Since it crosses the placenta it may lead to birth defects in baby. However, FDA research shows that most fish do not contain levels of mercury high enough to warrant concern over eating them in moderate amounts. The 2015 Dietary Guidelines for Americans recommends that women who are pregnant or breast-feeding should consume at least 8 and up to 12 ounces of a variety of seafood weekly, avoiding only four types of high-mercury fish: shark, tilefish, king mackerel, and swordfish.

## DO eat these superfoods.

Maximizing nutrients during pregnancy is majorly important since you really aren't adding too many additional calories, so each one needs to deliver potent nutrition. These foods all deliver multiple pregnancy benefits, and they will make your taste buds happy.

Eggs: Eggs are one of the best sources of choline, an essential mineral that works with folic acid to reduce the risk for neural tube defects and plays a role in your baby's brain health. Mom's intake of choline during pregnancy directly affects baby's brain development and function! In addition, eggs deliver low-fuss protein to meals and snacks. You can't get much easier than noshing on a hard-boiled egg. Also try the Shakshuka with Chickpeas and Feta (page 114) and the Potato Benedict (page 60) recipes, which both highlight eggs.

Dark Leafy Greens: While the nutritional details of each type of dark, leafy green differ, they do all share a few major nutrients. Vitamins A and C, potent antioxidants, are found in all the dark, leafy greens and help with keeping cells healthy. Vitamin K is essential for proper blood clotting and preventing excessive bleeding, and folate is involved in the formation of red blood cells and the formation of the neural tube. Many leafy greens also contain calcium and potassium, both of which can help prevent cramps. Nosh on dark leafies in meals like Chicken and Barley with Kale-Walnut Pesto (page 95) and the Loaded Fries (page 97).

Avocado: Avocado is a rich source of fat and also contains fiber, a combination that is especially satisfying. These green fruits also contain important pregnancy nutrients like folate, vitamin K, and vitamin C. They also pack in potassium, which can help reduce fluid retention. In addition, they're easy to use and add a smooth texture to a wide range of meals and snacks . . . they can even be used in sweet or savory dishes! Try avocado in the Twice-Baked Avocado Potatoes (page 113) and the Avocado Toast (page 43) recipes.

**Pumpkin Seeds:** These seeds contain an assortment of nutrients that help support the muscular changes your body goes through during pregnancy. Phosphorous, magnesium, and potassium can all be found in pumpkin seeds and can help prevent muscle cramps as well as aid in healthy muscle function as your muscles are stretched and asked to carry more weight. These seeds also provide a vegetarian source of iron and deliver zinc, a key nutrient in healing and repair. Pumpkin seeds are a star of the Orange and Pumpkin Seed Spinach Salad (page 52).

**Salmon:** Salmon delivers a powerful dose of docosahexaenoic acid (DHA), an omega-3 fatty acid. A developing baby's brain requires 50 to 70 mg of DHA each day during the third trimester for optimal growth and that DHA comes from mom's diet. This omega-3-rich fish also delivers protein and vitamin D, two other very important nutrients for both mom and baby. The Crunchy Salmon Salad Wrap (page 63) and the 10-Minute Maple-Mustard Salmon (page 150) both creatively feature this nutrient-packed fish.

**Yogurt:** Calcium needs don't increase during pregnancy, but unlike other vitamins and minerals, if you don't get enough from your diet or supplements, baby takes what he or she needs from your bones! Calcium is important to developing strong bones and teeth (for you and baby) as well as maintaining normal muscle contraction, blood clotting, and heart rhythm. Women typically fall short of daily calcium needs, and just 1 cup of low-fat plain (doctor it up with fresh fruit!) yogurt delivers nearly half a day's worth. Yogurt also contains probiotics, good bacteria that are being linked to everything from better digestion to improved immunity. Rock your taste buds with the Banana Bread–Yogurt Parfait (page 61) and the Orange-Carrot Cream Smoothie (page 109).

**Quinoa:** This ancient grain (actually a seed!) is a nutrition powerhouse that serves double duty as a whole grain and a good source of quality protein. This is super helpful if and when your usual animal-based sources of protein are making your stomach turn. It's also got fiber to help keep constipation away, folate to prevent neural tube defects, and iron to help meet your increased needs. The Veggie Stir-Fried Quinoa (page 49) or the Creamy Quinoa-Flaxseed Cereal with Strawberries and Coconut (page 180) are two of the several recipes that highlight this versatile ingredient.

Oats: This popular breakfast food is a healthy, whole grain carbohydrate choice that offers up fiber, B vitamins, and iron all at once. There are also anecdotal claims that eating oatmeal and other foods made with oats can give your milk supply a boost once baby is born. And although there's no scientific evidence to support this role, many women (and lactation consultants!) swear by it. We say it's worth a try since oats provide so many additional health benefits!

Strawberries: These berries shine for their combination of vitamin C, an antioxidant that can help your body absorb iron, and fiber (3 g/cup) to help keep things moving along. As a bonus, they contribute to your hydration! Eat them fresh or frozen and try them out in our yummy Strawberry-Chia Pudding Breakfast Pops (page 160) or in Crispy French Toast Fingers with Creamy Strawberry-Chia Dipping Sauce (page 123).

Beans: We're talking black beans, kidney beans, white beans, soy beans (edamame), pinto beans, chickpeas (garbanzo beans), and black-eyed peas. All beans are an excellent source of both types of fiber (soluble and insoluble), which means if you eat beans regularly you're less likely to suffer from extreme constipation, which can also lead to hemorrhoids (ouch!). Plus, beans pack in protein and other key pregnancy nutrients such as iron, folate, calcium, and zinc. You'll find beans in a variety of recipes in this book, from the Fennel and White Bean Salad (page 76) to the Asparagus and White Bean Strata (page 90), and the Chicken and Pinto Bean Nachos (page 131).

Walnuts: These tasty nuts are a plant/vegetarian source of omega-3 fatty acids, which are important to baby's brain development. While the type of omega-3s in walnuts isn't as readily available to the body as the type in seafood, they still contribute to your overall requirements and are healthful fats to include in your diet. Plus, walnuts are also a good source of magnesium and phosphorous. Whip up the Date-Nut Breakfast Bars (page 179) or the Chicken and Barley with Kale-Walnut Pesto (page 95).

# seven VIP nutrients for pregnancy

Your body utilizes many nutrients from food that play a role in growing a baby that is healthy and strong. These five are of extra importance because they're needed in greater amounts while you're pregnant, are essential to preventing birth defects, and/or are typically nutrients that many women don't get enough of.

## CALCIUM

Calcium is important for developing strong bones and teeth (for you and baby) as well as maintaining normal muscle contraction, blood clotting, and heart rhythm. Women typically meet only about 75% of their calcium needs. If you don't get enough from your diet or supplements, baby takes what he or she needs from your bones!

**AMOUNT**
Pregnancy and lactation: 1000 mg/day

**WHERE TO GET IT**
Food: Low-fat dairy products like 1% or skim milk, low-fat yogurt, and low-fat cheese.

Other sources: sesame seeds, tofu, broccoli, canned salmon with bones; fortified foods (orange juice, non-dairy milks, breakfast cereals, and cereal bars).

Supplements: Recommended if you do not consume enough dairy products or fortified foods.

## VITAMIN D

Without this vitamin, your body (and baby's) can't use calcium. Recent research also shows that vitamin D is vital to genetic imprinting, which may affect your baby's susceptibility to chronic disease later in life. Although vitamin D is made in your skin through exposure to UV light, research shows most people living in northern latitudes don't make enough throughout the year to meet their needs.

**AMOUNT**
Pregnancy and lactation: 1000 IU/day

**WHERE TO GET IT**
Food: Vitamin D fortified milk, salmon, some brands of yogurt (read the label), and some mushrooms.

Supplements: Many calcium supplements also contain vitamin D, as does your prenatal vitamin—but an additional supplement may be needed.

## IRON

Iron is needed to produce red blood cells and transport oxygen throughout the body. During pregnancy, you are producing more blood and iron needs increase. It's especially important to get enough iron while pregnant because your baby will need to store enough iron to last through their first few months after birth!

**AMOUNT**
Pregnancy: 30 mg/day  (You need supplemental iron in addition to eating iron-rich foods.)
Lactation: 9mg/day

**WHERE TO GET IT**
Food: Lean red meat, fish, poultry, dried fruits, iron-fortified cereals, and dried beans and peas.

Supplements: Look for a prenatal vitamin that contains 30mg of iron (Fe).

## PROTEIN

Protein contains amino acids, which are essential building blocks for human tissue. Adequate protein helps maximize fetal brain development, particularly in the last trimester. It also protects against pregnancy complications such as pre-eclampsia and poor placental function.

**AMOUNT**
Pregnancy: About 60 g/day  Carrying twins: 75 g/day
Lactation: 65 g/day

**WHERE TO GET IT**
Food: Lean meat, poultry, and fish; dried beans, nuts, eggs, cheese, and dairy products.

Supplements: Usually there's no need for shakes, bars, or other protein supplements.

## FOLIC ACID

Folic acid is a B vitamin that is involved in fetal cell division. Getting enough folic acid during your first trimester is extremely important for preventing birth defects called neural tube defects. Later in pregnancy, folic acid is important for the formation of red blood cells (yours and baby's).

**AMOUNT**
Pregnancy: 600 mcg total (400 mcg from fortified foods and/or supplements and 200 mcg from food)
Lactation: 500 mcg

**WHERE TO GET IT**
Food: Leafy greens, legumes, citrus fruits and juices, and whole wheat bread.

Synthetic sources: Fortified foods like breakfast cereals or other grains; supplements like prenatal vitamins.

## DHA

An essential fatty acid important for the development of baby's brain and vision. A developing baby's brain requires 50 to 70 mg of DHA each day during the third trimester for optimal growth and that DHA comes from mom's diet (mom needs to eat an average of 200 mg/day to meet mom and baby's requirements).

**AMOUNT**
Pregnancy and lactation: 200 mg/day

**WHERE TO GET IT**
Food: Wild salmon (fresh, canned), herring, mackerel (not king), sardines, anchovies, tuna, trout, Pacific oysters, omega-3–fortified eggs, ground flaxseed, walnuts, seaweed, walnut oil, canola oil, and soybeans.

## CHOLINE

Choline is an essential nutrient, meaning your body can't make it on its own. It is the building block for acetylcholine, a neurotransmitter involved in memory. The bonus is, not only can it be good for your brain to get enough choline, it also plays a role in baby's brain development, as researchers suggest women can boost the cognitive function of their baby by getting enough choline.

**AMOUNT**
Pregnancy: 450 mg/day
Lactation: 550 mg/day

**WHERE TO GET IT**
Food: Egg yolks, beef, milk, soybeans, citrus, wheat germ, and nuts.

# Setting Up the Ultimate Healthy, Happy Pregnancy Kitchen

Cooking at home is one of the best things you can do for yourself and your growing family in terms of nutrition. Sure, dining out can be fun, but you don't know exactly what is going into your food (hint: it's usually a lot more butter and salt than you'd ever think to add at home), the portions are giant, and you can't always customize what you order. The other benefit to preparing meals at home is that you have ingredients around on a regular basis, which means that when you're hungry at 4 p.m. on a Saturday, there actually is something to eat.

## why make more meals at home?

- **You know what's in your food:** Restaurants are notorious for adding a whole lot of salt, butter, and sugar to foods to add flavor. In your kitchen, you can use herbs and spices and measure the amount of salt to add flavor without copious amounts of sodium.

- **Better-quality ingredients:** When you're in your own kitchen, you can trust that the ingredients that you put into dishes are fresh. And if eating locally or using mostly organic ingredients is important to you, cooking at home ensures that's exactly what will be served.

- **There's less wait time:** In the time it takes to get ready, drive to a restaurant, sit down and order, and then wait for your food to arrive, you could be finished with a home-cooked meal.

- **The decisions are easier:** While looking over all the choices on the menu can be really fun, it can also derail goals to eat more fruits and veggies, and can end up creating situations where you eat much heavier food than you'd intended.

- **Fewer calories:** While pregnancy is not the time to diet, it is a time when keeping your weight gain to healthy levels can increase the health of you and baby, can make labor and delivery go more smoothly, and can make recovery from labor and delivery much more pleasant.

## Step 1: Give Your Fridge a Makeover

While it sounds like the ultimate pain in the booty, cleaning out and organizing your fridge actually saves a lot of time. In other words, put an hour into cleaning and organizing your fridge now and reap the benefits for months to come. When your fridge is organized and not crowded with old condiment bottles and stuff you never use, it's easier to find the ingredients you need to whip up a meal or snack. Follow these steps to a fridge that makes you smile when you open it. Or at least doesn't make you sigh and immediately close it.

1. **Out with the old:** Toss out condiments that have expired, never get used, or those that just take up space and hide stuff you actually might want to use. Once you've weeded through the condiments, get rid of other expired food, rotting food (we all have those forgotten foods at the back of the fridge or the bottom of a drawer), and items that you just don't eat.

2. **Clean up on aisle 2:** Off smells and spills can be a sign of bacteria breeding grounds and can turn you off to eating what's in your fridge. Remove all items from your fridge and give the shelves, drawers, and walls a good scrub with safe DIY cleaning supplies. We're big believers in using non-toxic cleaners in the kitchen. Our motto: Don't spray it near food or dishes if it's not safe to eat. Mix up a batch of our all-purpose kitchen cleaner for counters, fridge shelves, and walls.

---

## safe diy cleaning supplies

**All-purpose kitchen cleaner:** 1 cup of vinegar, 1 tablespoon of liquid soap, and 3 cups of water. Pour into a reusable spray bottle (find one at any Home Depot, Target, Wal-Mart, or plant supply store). For added fresh scent, add 4 to 6 drops of an essential oil (we love lemon, grapefruit, or lavender).

**Glass cleaner:** Mix 1 cup of grain alcohol, ¼ cup of white vinegar, ¼ teaspoon of liquid soap, and ½ gallon of water in a bucket. Pour into a reusable spray bottle and store the rest in a clean, well-labeled container with a tight-fitting lid. An empty plastic vinegar jug works well for storing any excess cleaner. Use to clean glass surfaces.

---

3. **Replace, reorganize:** When you reload your fridge, group like items together so they're easy to find. Stash dairy products in one section, refrigerated veggies in another, and leftovers in another. Make sure to use the "First In First Out" (FIFO) method when adding new foods to the fridge. Nothing like an acronym to really get this kitchen cleaning party started! FIFO means placing newer items behind older items, so the older ones get used first.

4. **What you see is what you eat:** Put easy-to-grab, ready-to-eat foods such as fruits and veggies (apples, baby carrots, celery sticks), yogurt, and hummus front and center in the fridge so they're the options you see first every time you open that door. Stash the foods that you don't want to eat as often (leftover birthday cake) closer to the back of the fridge or in the crisper drawers along with the veggies and fruit that you plan to use for meals and want to keep nice and crisp. If you're struggling to get enough fruit and veggies each day, putting those at eye level in the front of the fridge is key.

5. **Store produce wisely:** Nothing is sadder than produce that goes bad before it has been eaten! The way you store your fresh fruits and veggies can have a big impact on how long it lasts. Here are some of the basics to help extend the life of your produce:

   - Keep refrigerated produce in perforated plastic bags or storage containers.

   - Store herbs such as mint, cilantro, and rosemary—as well as asparagus—with the ends in a shallow glass or bowl of water like a bouquet (An 8-ounce juice glass or jar filled halfway works great.) Then cover with a plastic bag.

Healthy, Happy Pregnancy Cookbook

# produce storage guide

Refrigerate: apples (when storing longer than one week), artichokes, asparagus, beets, broccoli, brussels sprouts, cabbage, carrots, cauliflower, celery, cherries, corn, grapes, green beans, green onions, herbs (except basil), leafy vegetables, leeks, lettuce, mushrooms, okra, peas, plums, radishes, spinach, sprouts, summer squash, yellow squash, zucchini

* blackberries, blueberries, raspberries, strawberries

Store on counter: apples (when storing less than one week), bananas, basil, cucumbers, eggplant, garlic, ginger, grapefruit, jicama, lemons, limes, mangoes, oranges, papayas, peppers, persimmons, whole pineapple, plantains, pomegranates, tomatoes, whole watermelon

*Refrigerate berries, unwashed, and arrange in a single layer with paper towels in between layers. Or, leave them in their original packaging, unwashed, removing any berries that contain mold, as they can contaminate the others.*

## interesting factoid

**Ethylene gas:**

Did you know that fruits and vegetables produce an odorless, harmless gas called ethylene that can speed up the ripening process of other fruits and veggies around them? All fruits and vegetables produce it, but some in greater quantities. Keep high ethylene–producing fruits and veggies away from your already-ripe produce to make it last longer. Or, use it to your advantage to speed up the ripening process of an unripe fruit, by pairing unripe fruit with high ethylene–producing fruit in a paper bag. For example, put a peach in a paper bag with an unripe avocado.

Some of the highest ethylene–producing fruits and veggies are:

apples, apricots, avocados, bananas, cantaloupe, figs, nectarines, peaches, pears, plums, tomatoes

## Step 2: Tackle the Pantry

Clean out. Throw out. Reorganize. The same process that you used for your fridge makeover in Step 1 applies to your pantry/food cabinets, too, with the following addition to the reorganization phase.

Friendly pairings: Now that you have all of the food from your pantry strewn out on your counter, put foods that you typically use together in groups, and put them in places that make sense strategically. For instance, group oils, vinegars, honey, and soy sauce together on a shelf, since you'll often use them together in preparing sauces and salad dressings.

## pantry partners

Store these food items together:

- Breakfast foods: Dried fruits, oats, and whole grain cereal.
- Dinner staples: Whole grains, pasta, canned tomatoes, canned beans.
- Snack components: Popcorn kernels, whole grain crackers, and other snack items.
- Flavor boosters: Oils, vinegars, honey, soy sauce, hot sauce.

*Note: Nuts and seeds should be stored in the fridge or freezer, which increases their shelf life considerably.*

## Step 3: Find a Home for the Rest of It

Save time prepping, cooking, and cleaning by storing utensils and other kitchen supplies in the areas that you use them most. For instance, keep your cutting boards and knives near one another because you'll always use them together. The more efficient you make your kitchen experience the more likely you are to cook at home. Plus, saving 10 minutes in the kitchen means more minutes that you have for yourself and is especially good practice for saving time when baby arrives!

Near your food preparation area, store:

- Cutting boards
- Knives
- Mixing bowls
- Measuring cups

Healthy, Happy Pregnancy Cookbook

Next to your stove and microwave, store:

- Mixing spoons, spatulas, tongs
- Meat thermometer
- Spice rack
- Storage containers (for leftovers)
- Pots and pans
- Baking sheets, muffin tins, roasting dishes

## What You Really Need

Chances are you already have a lot of the kitchen stuff you need. In reality, you probably have WAY more than you need, evident by that drawer that everyone in your house refers to as "the junk drawer." We all have one, but consider paring down the stuff in your kitchen that you don't use, to free up space and to streamline your cooking process.

## Kitchen Tools

Here's what you need to have in your kitchen to make cooking at home a breeze. This list doesn't include eating utensils like forks, spoons, plates, bowls, chopsticks, and straws. We assume you know that those are a given (unless you're planning to eat with your hands—and in that case, you do you, girl!).

### 11 Must-have Kitchen Tools

1. Oven or toaster oven
2. Microwave
3. Stove-top range or electric burner (hot plate)
4. One 8- or 10-inch cast-iron or stainless steel skillet
5. Medium saucepan (about 1.5 quarts/6 cups) and lid
6. 8-inch chef's knife
7. Handheld immersion blender or standing blender
8. Two cutting boards: One for vegetarian fare; one for raw meat, poultry, and fish
9. One set of mixing bowls (at least three different sizes)
10. Baking sheet or shallow baking dish
11. Meat thermometer

How to use a meat thermometer:

- The thickest part of what you're measuring the temperature of will always be the last to reach the desired temperature—so measure that part.
- If you're cooking something with bones still in it, be sure not to let the thermometer touch the bone. Bone conducts heat faster and you'll get a falsely high reading.
- Wash the thermometer with soap and water every single time you use it. Otherwise you're poking raw meat germs into cooked meat!

Cooking temperatures (not too hot, not too cold, but juuuust right!):

- Pork, beef, veal, lamb: Cook to 145°F and let rest 3 minutes before serving.
- Ground meat (burgers, etc.): 160°F
- Poultry (including ground turkey or chicken burgers): 165°F

---

# fact or myth:

## Color is the best indicator of when meat/poultry is done cooking

MYTH! Using the "color test" doesn't tell you much about whether your meat/poultry is, in fact, cooked to a safe temperature. Meat that's still pink may be cooked to a safe temperature, while browned meat doesn't necessarily indicate it's cooked enough. Using a meat thermometer is key, not only for making sure your food is cooked enough, but also for ensuring that you're not OVER cooking it either. Say buh-bye to rubbery, dry chicken!

---

## "Nice-To-Have" Kitchen Tools

These aren't essential, but they're tools we love because they make the job easier! If you're on a budget, stock up on them as you can.

1. Glass or BPA-free plastic lunch/refrigerator storage containers with lids
2. Grill pan: stove-top grill pan or an electric grill (such as the George Foreman grill)
3. Dutch oven and/or soup pot with a lid
4. Food processor (mini or regular)
5. Different sized skillets (we love having one 8-inch and one 10- to 12-inch, or 15-inch for larger jobs.)
6. Refillable olive oil spray container, like the Misto
7. Teakettle

---

# meet the misto

Remember the squirt guns you'd pump up to get a powerful stream of water? Translate that pump-and-spray system to a small canister that holds olive oil and you've got the Misto, one of our kitchen staples. Fill the container with your preferred cooking oil (we like olive or sunflower), twist on the spray top, and then pump the whole thing up with the lid. You get a fine mist of spray, like store-bought cooking sprays, but you can use your favorite oil AND there's nothing to throw away when it's empty—you refill it! Grab your own Misto at Bed, Bath & Beyond or Amazon.com.

---

# Healthy Happy Pregnancy Cooking School: The Essentials

You don't have to be super knowledgeable and experienced in the kitchen to cook tasty meals, but you do need a little knowledge and some very basic skills. The truth is, once you've got the RIGHT skills, you can whip up tasty meals in no time and with little effort. Read the next few pages and bookmark them for future reference. The following info gives you everything you need to know to put together delicious, healthy, balanced meals.

## Roasted Veggies

You can roast just about any vegetable and expect a sweeter and more concentrated flavor that's sure to please even the most stubborn veggie eaters (or non-eaters). The high heat used in roasting caramelizes the natural sugars in the vegetables, taming the bitterness that often deters people from liking them. And it couldn't be simpler—unless someone else were cooking for you . . . All you need is a baking dish or rimmed baking sheet, olive oil, the vegetables that you're roasting, and any herbs or spices that you like.

1. Wash and scrub (or peel) vegetables.

2. Cut into equal-size pieces. Depending on the veggie, this might be ½- to 1-inch-square chunks or long and narrow strips. The size ultimately depends on what you'll be using the veggies for and what you prefer.

3. Place the cut veggies in a pile on the baking sheet/dish that you plan to cook them on. Coat with 1 teaspoon of olive oil per 1 cup of vegetables, about 1 tablespoon per pound.

4. Add any herbs, spices, or flavorings of choice. Some basic pairings are listed in the roasting chart, but don't be afraid to get creative!

5. Toss all the veggies together so that they're evenly coated with oil and flavorings. Spread out the veggies evenly on the baking sheet/dish, making sure not to overlap the pieces or they will steam instead of brown.

6. Bake at 400° to 425°F for 15 to 30 minutes, turning halfway through the baking time, until the vegetables are slightly browned on the outside and soft on the inside. Since not all veggies have the same cooking times and temps, use the handy guide on pages 24–25.

| Veggie | Amount | Size of pieces | Cooking temp./ time* | Flavor ideas (Choose one or more) |
|---|---|---|---|---|
| Asparagus | 1 pound; 20 medium/thick stalks or 40 thin stalks | Whole or halved spears | 400°F/15 minutes | Salt, pepper, ginger, garlic powder |
| Broccoli/ Cauliflower | 1 pound; 1 head/ bunch; 3 to 4 heaping cups chopped | 1-inch florets | 425°F/15–20 minutes | Salt, pepper, garlic powder, curry powder, lemon pepper |
| Brussels sprouts | 1 pound; 20 Brussels sprouts; 4 heaped cups of halved sprouts | Remove outer leaves, trim stem; halve lengthwise or leave whole if small | 425°F/20–25 minutes | Salt, pepper, honey, balsamic vinegar |
| Butternut squash | 2¼ pounds; 1 medium squash (8–10 inches long), 3½ heaping cups cubed | Peel and remove seeds, then cut into 1-inch cubes OR bake entire squash, whole, removing seeds and scooping out flesh after baking | 450°F/25–30 minutes | Cinnamon, pumpkin pie spice, salt, curry powder, cumin |
| Carrots/Parsnips | 1 pound; 1 bunch carrots; 6 medium carrots/parsnips | 1-inch pieces or ¼-inch-wide French fry-like strips | 425°F/20–25 minutes | Salt, pepper, garlic powder, paprika, oregano, rosemary |

| Veggie | Amount | Size of pieces | Cooking temp./ time* | Flavor ideas (Choose one or more) |
|---|---|---|---|---|
| Eggplant | 1½ pounds; 1 medium (8–10 inches long); 6 heaping cups cubed | 1-inch cubes, ½-inch slices, or cut in half lengthwise with shallow slits, cut cross-wise | 425°F, 20–30 minutes (use longer time for eggplant halves) | Garlic powder, salt, pepper |
| Fennel | 1½ pounds; 1 large bulb; 2 heaping cups sliced | Trim stalks and fronds (the hairy things) from the bulb, cut into 1-inch wedges | 450°F, 25–35 minutes | Salt, pepper |
| Green beans | 1 pound; 3½ heaped cups | whole, ends trimmed | 400°F/15–20 minutes | Salt, pepper, ginger, garlic powder |
| Peppers | 1½ pounds; 3 large peppers; 1½ cups chopped | 1-inch x 2-inch strips | 450°F, 25 minutes | Salt, pepper |
| Potatoes, red/ yukon gold | 1 pound; 1 large Russet (6 inches long); 20 fingerling; 6 red | 1-inch pieces or wedges, or thin French fry-like strips | 450°F/25–35 minutes | Garlic powder, paprika, pepper, cumin |
| Sweet potatoes | 1¼ pounds; 1 large potato (6 inches long) | 1-inch pieces or wedges, or thin French fry-like strips | 425°F/20–25 minutes | Chili powder, cinnamon, honey |

## Whole Grains

There's more to whole grains than brown rice and whole wheat bread—and, if you haven't tried many of the other options, you're missing out on awesome flavors, textures, and nutrition. Plus, many of them are just as convenient to make as pasta.

Whole grains are an important part of the Healthy, Happy Pregnancy lifestyle because they're an unrefined, fiber-rich source of carbohydrates. They are digested more slowly and spike your blood sugar less than refined grains, which is a good thing when it comes to keeping your energy level high and preventing gestational diabetes.

### Whole Grain Cooking Guide

| Grain | Taste/Texture | Uses | Cooking Instructions Ratio of grain: liquid + cooking time | Amount Cooked |
|-------|---------------|------|-----------------------------------------------------------|---------------|
| Amaranth | Fluffy, slightly sticky texture and mild popcorn taste | Pasta alternative, soup/stew addition, hot breakfast cereal | 1 cup : 3 cups 15–20 minutes | 2½ cups |
| Barley, hulled | Creamy taste and chewy texture | Warm or cold salads, soup/stew addition, pilaf | 1 cup : 3 cups 40–60 minutes | 3½ cups |
| Brown rice | Slightly chewy, with a warm, nutty flavor | Stir-fry, burrito filling, hot/cold breakfast cereal | 1 cup : 2 cups 40–50 minutes | 3–4 cups |
| Bulgur wheat | Very light, fluffy texture and mild flavor | Warm/cold salads, pilaf, hot/cold breakfast cereal | 1 cup : 2 cups 10–12 minutes | 3 cups |
| Millet | Fluffy texture with a buttery taste | Pasta alternative, soup/stew addition, salad addition, hot breakfast cereal | 1 cup : 2½ cups 25–35 minutes | 4 cups |

| Grain | Taste/Texture | Uses | Cooking Instructions Ratio of grain: liquid + cooking time | Amount Cooked |
|---|---|---|---|---|
| Quinoa | Slightly chewy texture with a bit of crunch and a mildly nutty flavor | Stir-fry, pilaf, pasta alternative, hot/cold breakfast cereal, soup/stew addition, side dish | 1 cup : 2 cups 12–15 minutes | 3–4 cups |
| Steel-cut oats | Chewier, heartier texture than rolled oats | Hot/cold breakfast cereal, in soups/stews | 1 cup : 4 cups 30 minutes | 3 cups |
| Wheat Berries | Subtle nutty flavor and chewy texture | Warm/cold salads, pilaf, hot/cold breakfast cereal, soup/stew addition, pasta alternative | 1 cup : 4 cups 45–60 minutes | 3 cups |
| Wild rice (actually a grass, not a rice!) | A little bit nutty and slightly chewy texture with long brown and/or black grains | Stir-fry, pilaf, stuffing for veggies | 1 cup : 3 cups 45–55 minutes | 3½ cups |

## key whole grain cooking points and instructions

- Most grains are cooked in a manner similar to rice. For the simplest method of cooking grains, combine the grain plus liquid (water, broth, or milk) in a saucepan and bring to a boil. Reduce the heat to low and simmer, covered, for the specified amount of time until most of the liquid has been absorbed; fluff with a fork.
- Even the same type of grain may have slightly different cooking times or liquid needs depending on its age, origin, and how it's been stored. Use the cooking times in the chart as a guide, but give your grains 5 to 10 minutes leeway in either direction.
- Whole grains keep well when stored in the fridge or frozen, so don't be afraid to make a bigger batch than you need at the time and freeze for later!

## more than one way to . . . cook a grain

- Creamy: Instead of water, cook the grain in milk and use as a breakfast cereal.
- Flavor boosted: Instead of water, cook the grain in low-sodium veggie or chicken broth.
- Pilaf style: Heat 1 teaspoon of oil and ½ cup of chopped onion for every cup of grain in the bottom of a saucepan until golden. Add the grain, stir, and sauté for 2 minutes, stirring continuously. Add water and cook per instructions. For a fruit and nut pilaf, stir ¼ cup of dried fruit and ¼ cup of chopped nuts/seeds into the cooked grain for every cup of dry grain used.

### Eggs

Eggs are back—yolk and all! And for good reason: Eggs are the complete nutrition package. They're inexpensive; packed with important pregnancy (and beyond) nutrients such as high-quality protein, choline, and vitamin D; and oh so versatile. In recent years, studies have also shown that eating eggs at breakfast time may help you control weight by quelling hunger. You'll find eggs in many of the recipes in this book.

Six Easy Ways to Cook Eggs

1. Hard-cooked: Place the eggs in a saucepan and cover with enough cool tap water to come an inch or two above the tops of the eggs. Place the saucepan over high heat and bring the water to a boil. Remove the saucepan from the burner and let sit, covered, for about 12 minutes (less time if you like your yolks moist). Or, put an egg (or several eggs) right onto the oven rack and bake at 425°F for 10 to 12 minutes. Remove with tongs or an oven mitt. Whether you cook them on the stove top or in the oven, rinse with cold water to stop the cooking process before eating or storing in the fridge.

---

### interesting factoid

**Why aren't they hard-BOILED eggs?**

Most of us call them hard-boiled eggs, but really hard-cooked is the way to go. You never want to cook eggs in boiling water because a greenish ring will form around the yolk (the result of components of the yolk interacting at the high temperature).

---

2. Soft-boiled: Bring a medium saucepan of water to a rolling boil over medium-high heat. Place an egg into the water, wait 30 seconds, then cover the pan and remove it from the heat. Let your egg sit in the hot water for 5 to 7 minutes. Rinse under cool water to stop the cooking process and serve.

3. Poached: Fill a medium saucepan two-thirds of the way with water and bring to a simmer (bubbles should be rising from the bottom to top, but not at a full boil). Add 1 tablespoon of vinegar. With a large spoon or ladle, stir the water quickly in a circle so that it forms a moving whirlpool. Crack a cold egg (straight from the fridge) into the center of the whirlpool. Allow the egg to simmer until the white and yolk are firm. Remove from the water with a slotted spoon, letting any excess water drain off.

4. Scrambled: Measure 1 tablespoon of 1% or skim milk (or water) for each egg you'll be using. Whisk the milk or water and eggs, and add a sprinkle of salt and pepper and any other herbs or spices you like. Heat ½ teaspoon of oil per egg in a skillet over medium-high heat and pour in the eggs. Don't stir the eggs—turn and fold them gently with a wooden spoon or spatula until just set.

5. Fried: Coat a skillet with cooking spray or coat with ½ teaspoon of olive oil or other vegetable oil and place over medium-high heat. Crack an egg open and let it slide onto the skillet. Reduce the heat to medium and cook for about 3 minutes, or until the white is firm and yolk begins to thicken. Flip the egg and cook an additional minute or two, or until the yolk is firm.

---

### interesting factoid

**Are runny egg yolks safe?**

Most of the time, yes, the risk is quite small. The major risk with undercooked egg yolks is salmonella. To best reduce your likelihood of becoming sick from this bacterium, both the white and yolk of an egg should be cooked until firm. Our recommendation is that pregnant women, young children, older adults, and people with weakened immune systems stick with well-cooked (totally firm) eggs.

---

6. Microwave scramble: Measure 1 tablespoon of 1% or skim milk (or water) for each egg and whisk or stir with a fork. Add a sprinkle of salt and pepper and any other favorite herbs or spices—we love a pinch of dried chili powder and garlic powder. Place in a microwave-safe mug or bowl and microwave on high for 1 minute. Stir and microwave for another 30 to 45 seconds (or skip the stirring to keep your eggs in the perfect shape to fit on an English muffin for an egg sandwich).

Healthy, Happy Pregnancy Cookbook

# Packaged Food Basics: What to Look For

For the most part, opting for the least processed foods you can find will make your overall diet healthier. But, sometimes packaged foods help to pull a healthy meal together and some packaged foods aren't actually processed in a detrimental way (for example, peanut butter or canned beans). Use these criteria to choose the most healthful versions of the many processed foods available.

### Almond/Peanut Butter (per 2 tablespoons)

- Almonds/peanuts and salt are the only ingredients

### Bagel (per bagel)

- 250 calories or less
- At least 4 g fiber
- No more than 450 mg sodium
- Whole grain is the first ingredient

### Bread (per slice)

- At least 3 g fiber
- No more than 160 mg sodium
- 100% whole grain
- No partially hydrogenated oils/trans fats

### Gluten-Free Bread (per slice)

- At least 2 g fiber
- No partially hydrogenated oils/trans fats
- No more than 160 mg sodium

### Gluten-Free Cereal (per ½ cup)

- No more than 6 g sugar
- At least 2 g fiber
- No more than 250 mg sodium per cup
- Whole grain is the first ingredient
- No partially hydrogenated oils/trans fats
- Must be produced in a gluten-free facility or verified to contain less than 20 parts per million (ppm) gluten

### Cereal (per ½ cup)

- No more than 6 g sugar
- At least 3 g fiber
- No more than 250 mg sodium per cup
- Whole grain is the first ingredient
- No partially hydrogenated oils/trans fats

### Crackers (per 1 ounce)

- No more than 1.5 g saturated fat
- At least 3 g fiber
- No more than 180 mg sodium
- No partially hydrogenated oils/trans fats
- Whole grain is the first ingredient

### Gluten-Free Crackers (per 1 ounce)

- No more than 1.5 g saturated fat
- At least 2 g fiber
- No more than 180 mg sodium
- No partially hydrogenated oils/trans fats
- A whole grain is the first ingredient
- Must be produced in a gluten-free facility or verified to contain less than 20 parts per million (ppm) gluten

### English Muffin (per muffin)

- 100% whole grain
- At least 3 g fiber
- No partially hydrogenated oil
- No high-intensity sweeteners*

### Snack Bar

- No partially hydrogenated oils/trans fats
- At least 5 g fiber
- No more than 4 g saturated fat
- At least 5 g protein
- Contains at least one of: whole grains, fruit, nuts
- No high-intensity sweeteners*

### Frozen Breakfast Sandwich or Wrap (per item)

- At least 3 g fiber
- No more than 5 g saturated fat
- At least 10 g protein
- No more than 500 mg sodium
- No partially hydrogenated oils

### Frozen Burrito (per burrito)

- At least 250 calories, no more than 500 calories
- 2 g saturated fat or less
- At least 4 g fiber
- At least 8 g protein
- 500 mg or less sodium
- No partially hydrogenated oils/trans fat
- No artificial flavors/preservatives

### Frozen Pizza (per serving)

- No more than 4.5 g saturated fat
- No more than 700 mg sodium
- At least 4 g fiber
- No partially hydrogenated oils/trans fats

### Frozen Gluten-Free Pizza (per serving)

- No more than 5 g saturated fat
- No more than 700 mg sodium
- At least 2 g fiber
- No partially hydrogenated oils/trans fats

Frozen Sweet Potato Fries (per 3 ounces)

- No more than 0.5 g saturated fat
- At least 2 g fiber
- No more than 200 mg sodium

Frozen Waffles (per 2 waffles)

- No more than 1 g saturated fat
- No more than 5 g sugar
- At least 3 g fiber
- No more than 360 mg sodium
- No partially hydrogenated oils/trans fats
- Whole grain is the first ingredient (or second ingredient after water)

Frozen Fruit Pop

- No more than 28 g sugar
- Ingredients list fruit before sugar
- No high-intensity sweeteners*

Granola (per ¼ cup)

- No more than 5 g sugar
- No high-intensity sweeteners*
- At least 2 g fiber
- No partially hydrogenated oils/trans fats

Chewy Granola Bar (per bar)

- No more than 1.5 g saturated fat
- No more than 9 g sugar
- At least 3 g fiber
- No partially hydrogenated oils/trans fats
- Whole grain/nuts/seeds are the first ingredients*
- No high-intensity sweeteners*

Crunchy Granola Bar (per bar)

- No more than 1.5 g saturated fat
- No more than 10 g sugar
- At least 3 g fiber
- No partially hydrogenated oils/trans fats
- Whole grain is the first ingredient
- No high-intensity sweeteners*

Hummus (per 2 tablespoons)

- 70 calories or less
- No more than 1 g saturated fat
- No more than 130 mg sodium
- No artificial preservatives (such as potassium sorbate)

Ice Cream (per ½ cup)

- No high-intensity sweeteners*
- No partially hydrogenated oils/trans fats

### Flavored Instant Oatmeal (per packet)

- No more than 5 g sugar per 100 calories
- At least 2 g fiber per 100 calories
- No more than 75 mg sodium per 100 calories
- Oats are the first ingredient
- No partially hydrogenated oils/trans fat
- No high-intensity sweeteners*

### Unsweetened Instant Oatmeal (per packet)

- At least 2 g fiber per 100 calories
- No more than 80 mg sodium per 100 calories
- Oats are the first ingredient
- No partially hydrogenated oils
- No sweeteners/high-intensity sweeteners added

### Pastas (per 2 ounces dry)

- At least 5 g fiber
- No added salt
- 100% whole grain

### Gluten-Free Pastas (per 2 ounces dry)

- At least 2 g fiber
- No added salt
- Must be produced in a gluten-free facility or verified to contain less than 20 parts per million (ppm) gluten

### Pasta Sauce (per ½ cup)

- No more than 0.5 g saturated fat
- No more than 400 mg sodium
- No more than 8 g sugar

### Salad Dressing (per 1 tablespoon)

- No more than 1 g saturated fat
- No more than 2.5 g sugar
- No more than 150 mg sodium
- No artificial flavors/natural flavors/ colors/preservatives or high-intensity sweeteners

### Salsa (per 2 tablespoons)

- 15 calories or less
- No more than 3 g sugar
- No more than 150 mg sodium

### Sorbet (per ½ cup)

- No more than 28 g sugar
- Ingredients list fruit before sugar
- No high-intensity sweeteners*

### Veggie Burger (per patty)

- No more than 1 g saturated fat
- At least 10 g protein
- No more than 350 mg sodium
- Uses non-GMO/organic soy

Whole Wheat Wrap/Tortilla
(per 6- to 8-inch wrap)

- At least 2 g fiber
- No more than 310 mg sodium
- Whole grain is the first ingredient
- No high-intensity sweeteners*
- No partially hydrogenated oil/trans fat

Plain Yogurt (per 6 ounces)

- Contains at least 25% of the RDA for calcium
- Uses milk not treated with rBGH

Flavored Yogurt (per 6 ounces)

- No more than 30 g sugar
- Contains at least 25% of the RDA for calcium
- Uses milk not treated with rBGH

*High-intensity sweeteners include artificial sweeteners, sugar alcohols, monk fruit extract, and stevia extract.

# are oats gluten-free?

Gluten is a protein found in wheat, rye, and barley, and sometimes oats. It's that caveat about oats that can be really confusing. The bottom line: Oats don't naturally contain gluten, but they're often grown near fields of grains that do, which can lead to gluten contamination of oats. The same goes for factories that process oats into the steel-cut or the rolled variety you cook up at home—some of them also process gluten-containing grains and this leaves room for cross-contamination. If you have celiac disease or gluten intolerance, opt for oats that specify that they are gluten-free and have been tested to ensure they do not contain any traces of gluten. It is rare, but possible, for people with celiac disease to be sensitive to a protein in oats (we're not sure the exact reason for this yet) that can cause a reaction similar to that of gluten. For this reason, the Academy of Nutrition and Dietetics (AND) suggests that up to ½ cup of gluten-free oats each day is generally safe for people who have celiac disease but that you should speak with your doctor if you notice reaction symptoms. The recipes in this book that use oats with no other gluten-containing ingredients are labeled as gluten-free, assuming that you use gluten-free oats.

# Healthy, Happy Pregnancy-Style Dining Out

Okay, okay! Cooking at home yields healthier meals that use better ingredients, but sometimes you just want to go out to eat. And there is nothing wrong with that. In fact, taking a night off from cooking can be just the ticket to a relaxing evening once in a while. Dining out doesn't have to mean excess sodium, fat, sugar, and portions if you follow these tips.

1. Do some research: Check out the menu online to see which dishes sound good, and, if you have any questions about the safety of ingredients (do they use unpasteurized cheeses, etc.), you can call ahead to ask.

2. Have a snack before you head out: Arriving to a restaurant when you're really hungry is a little bit like walking by a sale right after you've been paid—everything seems like a good choice. You're much more likely to make a nutritious choice, eat slowly, and stop eating when you're satisfied but not overly stuffed if you've had a pre-dinner snack. Plus, your dinner companions might enjoy you a bit more if you don't arrive all "hangry."

3. Be realistic about frequency and occasion: If you rarely dine out and this is your partner's birthday dinner, go a little crazy if you feel like it. Start with an appetizer. Have a heavier dish. Share dessert. But if you dine out on a regular basis, then there are just too many opportunities for special occasion eating. So, if you're a frequent restaurant-goer, make a balanced, nutritious choice even for special occasions. And no matter what the occasion, respect your body's fullness cues and stop before you're stuffed.

4. Skip the chips (and bread, bread sticks, and crackers): The foods that restaurants often put out, like chips or a bread bowl, are typically more processed and less nutritious. Skip them and save your precious stomach space for foods that pack in nutrition.

5. Ask for what you want: Don't feel embarrassed about ordering food exactly the way you want it—it's your meal, your money, and your health. Speak up if you have questions about the safety of ingredients or how things are cooked. And if you want to switch an ingredient from one dish to another, ask! The worst that can happen is that they'll tell you it can't be done. Best case scenario is you get a totally perfectly awesome meal.

6. Share: Sharing an entrée and a few sides or two entrées or an entrée and an app, etc., is a great way to get a variety of flavors and more nutrition. Plus, it's a fun way to keep tabs on portions.

## food tips by food type

Salads: Swap croutons with beans, order dressing on the side and use 2 spoonfuls, and ask for plain chopped nuts in lieu of candied nuts.

Burgers: Ask for a whole grain bun and that it not be toasted with butter (a common restaurant practice), and opt for a side salad or side of steamed veggies.

Burritos: Opt for beans or chicken/beef/pork/tofu as your filling with veggies instead of rice, skip sour cream and opt for salsa, consider a burrito bowl made with beans or brown rice as the base for the fillings instead of a tortilla.

# A Note About Special Diet Icons

We know that one size does not fit all when it comes to special diet preferences and needs. For this reason, we created special diet icons to make finding the right recipe at the right time even easier. The icons that you see before each recipe are there to quickly let you know if the recipe meets specific diet criteria (i.e., gluten-free), provides a substantial amount of a VIPN (very important pregnancy nutrient), and/or is super-fast to make. While leafing through recipes, and glancing at the nutrition information provided, you'll notice that each recipe provides a variety of nutrients and that many of the important pregnancy nutrients, are abundant. We used a variety of less refined, whole food ingredients to ensure that the recipes provide high-quality nutrition, and lots of nutrient variety.

You'll also notice that not every nutrient or positive recipe attribute is called out with diet icons—if we did this, this book would be ten billion (mild exaggeration) pages long. Instead, the diet icons indicate recipes that meet many of the most common (and often requested) dietary constraints (gluten-free, dairy-free, and vegetarian), recipes that deliver a powerful amount of the VIPNs that are commonly low in women's diets (fiber, iron, and calcium), and super-speed recipes that take 20 minutes or less to make (everyone needs those!).

Here's the guide to what these labels mean.

 **GLUTEN-FREE:** Free of any gluten-containing ingredients.

 **VEGETARIAN:** No meat, poultry, or fish.

 **DAIRY-FREE:** Free of any dairy and dairy-containing products.

 **FIBER-RICH:** At least 5 mg fiber per serving (20% Daily Value).

 **IRON-RICH:** At least 3.6 mg iron per serving (20% Daily Value).

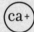 **CALCIUM-RICH:** At least 200 mg calcium per serving (20% Daily Value).

 **FAST RECIPE:** Takes 20 minutes or less to make, from start to finish.

## a note on folate and folic acid

You may notice that we didn't report folate (the food form of this important pregnancy B vitamin) in the nutrition information or diet notes. The recipes do include many foods high in folate, like leafy greens and legumes, making many of the recipes a good source of this nutrient. However, folic acid, the synthetic version of this nutrient, is found in adequate amounts in your prenatal vitamin. This is why we didn't report exact amounts for each recipe. In other words, eating foods rich in folate is important and these recipes provide a lot, but your needs for that nutrient will also be met by your prenatal vitamin.

# I'm Gonna Hurl . . . But I'm Still Hungry: Recipes to Ease Nausea

Nausea sucks. There's really no other way to put it that fully captures the "suckiness." And what is often referred to as morning sickness is not confined to first thing in the morning—"morning" sickness can come on during that pre-lunch office meeting, while out shopping on a weekend afternoon, or during your commute home from work. So, let's just refer to this as nausea, with no time of day stipulation, from here on out.

The good news is that there are things you can do to reduce the chances of getting nauseated in the first place, as well as the severity when you are. Most important, do not let yourself get too hungry. In that sense, every chapter in this book is an anti-nausea chapter. Make sure you have a snack in your purse at all times (we've got you covered with some portable ideas) so that you don't get to the stomach-rumbling point. More specific to this chapter are the practices of ensuring you are getting enough protein at every meal and snack, including ginger and foods rich in vitamins $B_6$ and $B_{12}$, and making foods the least offensive they can be. In other words, this chapter provides you with foods that won't smell up the house when you prep them, and includes ingredients that will help ward off or reduce nausea.

# Pineapple-Kiwi Green Machine Smoothie

A cold, refreshing smoothie can be just the ticket when you're feeling queasy in the morning (or anytime, really). This smoothie not only provides great flavor, but it also delivers a hefty dose of protein and veggies—two things that might be lacking in your diet when you're nauseated.

makes 2 servings / prep time: 5 minutes / total time: 5 minutes

**2½ cups frozen pineapple chunks**

**2 very ripe kiwi fruit, washed but not peeled, hard end piece removed, sliced**

**2 cups skim milk or unsweetened dairy-free alternative**

**2 cups baby spinach**

**½ cup soft or silken tofu**

**⅓ cup full-fat canned coconut milk**

**1 cup ice cubes**

Combine the pineapple, kiwi, skim milk, spinach, tofu, and cocnut milk in a blender and blend on high until smooth, about 1½ minutes. Add the ice and blend again until all the ice is incorporated, about 1 minute more.

Per serving: 341 calories, 15 g protein, 52 g carbohydrates, 5.7 g fiber, 39 g total sugar, 11 g fat, 7.5 g saturated fat, 164 mg sodium, 1210 mg potassium (35% DV), 609 mg calcium (60% DV), 121 mg magnesium (30% DV), 0.939 mcg B12 (16% DV), 0.439 mg B6 (22% DV), 3.4 mg iron (19% DV)

# Avocado Toast

If you're craving carbs first thing in the a.m., this avocado toast will become your best friend. The lime juice adds a refreshing flavor, the avocado delivers healthy fats, and the whole grain toast boasts B vitamins that can help ease nausea.

makes 1 serving / prep time: 5 minutes / total time: 5 minutes

½ teaspoon olive oil

2 slices whole grain bread

¾ ripe avocado

1 teaspoon freshly squeezed lime juice

⅛ teaspoon coarse sea salt, divided

2 pinches chili powder or smoked paprika

Heat the oil in a medium skillet over medium heat. Toast the bread until golden and crispy on both sides, about 5 minutes total. Or toast the bread in a toaster until golden.

Mash the avocado, lime juice, and ¼ teaspoon of the salt together until only small lumps remain.

Spread the avocado mixture onto the toast and top each with a pinch of chili powder and the remaining ¼ teaspoon salt.

Per serving: 391 calories, 2 g protein, 50 g carbohydrates, 16 g fiber, 4 g total sugar, 21 g fat, 3.5 g saturated fat, 402 mg sodium, 547 mg potassium (16% DV), 101 mg calcium (10% DV), 34 mg magnesium (9% DV), 0 mcg B12 (0% DV), 0.319 mg B6 (16% DV), 3.2 mg iron (18% DV)

# Apple Pie Teff Hot Cereal

It's not always easy to stomach protein-rich foods first thing in the morning when you're battling nausea. This recipe will not only become one of your family staples because it's so delicious (hot cereal and your grandma's apple crumble had a baby and this is it) but it's also naturally got a hefty dose of protein and nausea-fighting B vitamins. If you've never seen teff in your local supermarket, look for the section where Bob's Red Mill brand products are sold. If it's not there, you can order it via Amazon.com. P.S. If you've ever had the Ethiopian bread injera, the grain used to make it is teff!

makes 4 servings / prep time: 5 minutes / total time: 35 minutes

1 cup teff or quinoa

4 cups skim milk or unsweetened soy milk

1 cup water

2 apples, cored and chopped, divided

½ teaspoon ground cinnamon

¼ cup chopped walnuts

8 teaspoons pure maple syrup

Pour the teff into a large saucepan and toast over medium-low heat, stirring with a spoon, until it begins to make a popping noise and smells like graham crackers, about 4 minutes.

Stir in the milk, water, half the chopped apples, and the cinnamon and bring to a boil. Once the mixture reaches a boil, reduce to a simmer, cover, and cook, stirring every 5 minutes to prevent it from sticking to the pan, until the teff is creamy and all the water has been absorbed, about 25 minutes. Watch it carefully so it doesn't simmer over, and stir with a large wooden spoon to prevent it from bubbling up and splashing your hand. This is where a very large saucepan comes in handy!

Divide the mixture among 4 bowls and top each with one-quarter of the remaining apples, 1 tablespoon of the walnuts, and 2 teaspoons of the maple syrup.

Per serving: 380 calories, 16 g protein, 67 g carbohydrates, 6 g fiber, 29 g total sugar, 6 g fat, 1 g saturated fat, 111 mg sodium, 722 mg potassium (21% DV), 414 mg calcium (41% DV), 133 mg magnesium (33% DV), 1.298 mcg B12 (22% DV), 0.392 mg B6 (20% DV), 4.2 mg iron (23% DV)

# Peach-Ginger Smoothie

    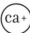 

A smoothie is a nauseated mom-to-be's best friend for several reasons. It can be made the night before so you don't even have to look at ingredients in the morning, it's cold and refreshing, and it's a simple way to pack lots of nutrition into a sipable package. The ginger in this smoothie can also help nix nausea, and, if you're not stomaching as many veggies as you did prepregnancy, this smoothie gives you a small boost.

makes 2 servings / prep time: 5 minutes / total time: 5 minutes

**3 very ripe peaches, or frozen and thawed (about 2 cups sliced)**

**1 large carrot, coarsely chopped**

**¾ cup skim milk or unsweetened dairy-free alternative**

**2 medium dried Medjool or Deglet Noor dates, pitted and chopped**

**3 tablespoons unsalted natural almond butter**

**½-inch piece fresh ginger, peeled and chopped**

**¼ teaspoon pure vanilla extract**

**¼ teaspoon ground turmeric**

**Pinch of ground cinnamon**

**1 cup ice cubes**

Add the peaches, carrot, milk, dates, almond butter, ginger, vanilla, turmeric, and cinnamon to a blender and puree on high until smooth, about 2 minutes. Add the ice and blend until incorporated, about 1 minute more.

Per serving: 320 calories, 11 g protein, 43 g carbohydrates, 8 g fiber, 34 g total sugar, 14 g fat, 1 g saturated fat, 75 mg sodium, 1006 mg potassium (29% DV), 303 mg calcium (30% DV), 109 mg magnesium (27% DV), 0.352 mcg B12 (6% DV), 0.195 mg B6 (10% DV), 1.8 mg iron (10% DV)

# Dried Plum (aka Prune) Muffins

Muffins can be such an easy way to fulfill major carb cravings in an easy to tote form. But, many are carb bombs that leave your blood sugar spiked and your energy level zapped shortly after eating. These muffins deliver protein and fiber to help sustain energy levels . . . and contain less sugar than a bite of many bakery muffins. They're also delicious. You're welcome.

makes 12 servings / prep time: 10 minutes + 30 minutes soak time / total time: 1 hour 20 minutes

1 cup dried pitted plums (prunes), divided

Cooking spray

1 (15-ounce) can white beans, rinsed and drained

2 large very ripe bananas

2 large eggs

2 tablespoons sunflower seed oil

¼ cup plus 2 tablespoons skim milk or unsweetened dairy-free alternative

2 teaspoons pure vanilla extract

½ cup old-fashioned rolled oats

1 cup almond meal

½ teaspoon baking soda

1½ teaspoons baking powder

½ teaspoon ground cinnamon

½ teaspoon ground ginger

¼ teaspoon ground cloves

½ cup roasted unsalted sunflower seeds

In a small bowl, soak ½ cup of the plums in warm water to cover for 30 minutes to soften.

Preheat the oven to 350°F. Line a 12-cup muffin tin with muffin wrappers and spray well with cooking spray.

Gently drain any excess water from the soaked plums and add to a blender or food processor with the beans, bananas, eggs, oil, milk, and vanilla. Puree on high until smooth, about 1 minute. Add the remaining ingredients except the sunflower seeds and the remaining ½ cup unsoaked plums. Puree on high until smooth, about 1 minute more. You may need to scrape down the sides of the blender to ensure even blending, as the mixture will be pretty thick.

Stir in the sunflower seeds. Pour the batter into the muffin tin, filling to the very top. Bake until the muffins are firm with golden tops, about 40 minutes. If the muffins are still soft in the centers, continue to bake in 5-minute increments until firm. Remove from the oven and allow to cool completely before serving. Store leftovers in the refrigerator.

Per serving: 280 calories, 11 g protein, 38 g carbohydrates, 8 g fiber, 10 g total sugar, 11 g fat, 1 g saturated fat, 133 mg sodium, 584 mg potassium (17% DV), 114 mg calcium (11% DV), 92 mg magnesium (23% DV), 0.141 mcg B12 (2% DV), 0.24 mg B6 (12% DV), 3.2 mg iron (18% DV)

Healthy, Happy Pregnancy Cookbook

# The Ultimate Chopped Salad

A chopped salad is tough to beat for a refreshing meal. And if you're one of the women who finds only raw veggies tolerable during the first trimester (or beyond), this will be a go-to recipe for you. Not only is it packed with crunchy, fresh veggies, but they're all in bite-size pieces so you don't have to worry about wrestling with a giant leaf of lettuce. This salad uses fresh herbs to deliver major flavor, and combines protein-rich chicken with high-fiber carbs from the potatoes to provide a balanced meal in a bowl.

makes 4 servings / prep time: 15 minutes / total time: 30 minutes

**5 medium red or purple potatoes (about 2¼ pounds)**

**1 teaspoon coarse sea salt, divided**

**16 ounces grilled chicken breast, chopped**

**2 large carrots, chopped into ¼-inch cubes**

**1 medium cucumber, chopped into ¼-inch cubes**

**4 plum tomatoes, seeded and chopped into ¼-inch cubes**

**6 large fresh basil leaves, finely chopped (or 1½ tablespoons dried)**

**4 fresh mint leaves, finely chopped, or 1 tablespoon dried**

**2 tablespoons olive oil**

**2 tablespoons balsamic vinegar**

**2 teaspoons Dijon mustard**

**¼ teaspoon freshly ground black pepper**

Add the potatoes and ½ teaspoon of the salt to a medium saucepan, cover by 1 inch with cold water, and bring to a boil. Reduce to a simmer and cook until the potatoes are tender, about 12 minutes. Drain and set aside to cool.

Toss the chicken, carrots, cucumber, tomatoes, basil, and mint in a large bowl. Whisk together the oil, vinegar, mustard, pepper, and remaining ½ teaspoon salt in a small bowl and pour over the salad. Toss to coat evenly. Cut the potatoes into 8 pieces each and add to the salad mixture. Toss very gently to incorporate potatoes without breaking them up.

Per serving: 449 calories, 37 g protein, 51 g carbohydrates, 7 g fiber, 9 g total sugar, 11 g fat, 2 g saturated fat, 412 mg sodium, 2081 mg potassium (% DV), 64 mg calcium (6% DV), 115 mg magnesium (29% DV), 0.284 mcg B12 (0% DV), 1.479 mg B6 (70% DV), 3 mg iron (17% DV)

# Quinoa-Veggie "Cheeseburgers"

Craving a cheeseburger but even the thought of the smell of cooking meat makes you a little barfy? This dish tastes like a cheeseburger but doesn't fill the house with the smell of cooking meat. And it delivers protein in addition to B vitamins, which might help soothe those "queasies."

makes 4 servings / prep time: 25 minutes / total time: 30 minutes

**2 tablespoons olive oil, divided**

**½ cup finely chopped cremini mushrooms**

**¼ cup finely chopped celery**

**¼ cup finely chopped onion**

**¼ cup finely chopped carrots**

**½ teaspoon coarse sea salt**

**¼ teaspoon garlic powder**

**⅛ teaspoon freshly ground black pepper**

**1 large egg, beaten**

**1½ cups cooked quinoa**

**3 tablespoons whole wheat flour**

**½ cup shredded cheddar cheese or dairy-free substitute**

Heat 1 tablespoon of the oil in a large skillet over medium heat. Add the mushrooms, celery, onion, and carrots and sauté until tender, 10 to 15 minutes. Remove the skillet from the heat and stir in the salt, garlic powder, and pepper.

Stir the egg and quinoa together in a medium bowl. Fold in the veggie mixture, stirring well to ensure the mixture is well combined. Stir in the flour and incorporate; then stir in the cheese. Using your hands, shape the quinoa mixture into 4 patties, 3 to 4 inches in diameter.

Heat the remaining 1 tablespoon oil in the same skillet over medium heat. Add the patties and cook until golden on both sides and firm, about 3 minutes on each side. Be careful when turning so they don't fall apart.

Per serving: 242 calories, 9 g protein, 20 g carbohydrates, 3 g fiber, 2 g total sugar, 14 g fat, 4.5 g saturated fat, 263 mg sodium, 256 mg potassium (7% DV), 130 mg calcium (13% DV), 59 mg magnesium (15% DV), 0.282 mcg B12 (5% DV), 0.168 mg B6 (8% DV), 1.6 mg iron (9% DV)

# Veggie Stir-Fried Quinoa

Who doesn't like a stir-fry? No one, that's who. But this stir-fry takes it to another level by acting as a sort of cross between fried rice and a quinoa bowl. It's easy to make, only dirties one dish in the process, and results in a meal that is packed with B vitamins, veggies, protein, and tummy-soothing ginger. Plus, it's another protein-rich meatless meal if meat isn't something you're feeling like eating right now. It's also a great one-container dish to take to work for lunch.

makes 4 servings / prep time: 10 minutes / total time: 25 minutes

1½ tablespoons sunflower seed oil (olive and coconut oil also work well)

1 (16-ounce) package extra-firm tofu, cubed

2½ cups snow peas or green beans

2 cups quartered cremini mushrooms

1 cup sliced carrots (cut about ¼ inch thick on the diagonal)

1 cup coarsely chopped bell peppers (1- to 2-inch chunks)

½ large yellow onion, chopped

⅓ cup vegetable broth

1 tablespoon grated fresh ginger

2 large garlic cloves, minced

3 tablespoons reduced-sodium soy sauce or gluten-free tamari

¼ cup rice vinegar

1 tablespoon toasted sesame oil

1 tablespoon ketchup

2 cups cooked quinoa

¼ teaspoon coarse sea salt

Heat the sunflower seed oil in a very large skillet or wok over medium heat. Add the tofu, peas, mushrooms, carrots, bell peppers, and onion and cook until the carrots are crisp-tender and the tofu is lightly browned, 15 to 20 minutes.

Add the broth, ginger, and garlic and simmer for 1 minute. Whisk together the soy sauce, vinegar, sesame oil, and ketchup and stir into the veggie mixture. Then stir in the quinoa. Cook until all the ingredients are heated through, about 4 minutes more. Sprinkle with the salt and serve.

Per serving: 373 calories, 18 g protein, 41 g carbohydrates, 7 g fiber, 9 g total sugar, 16 g fat, 1.5 g saturated fat, 618 mg sodium, 640 mg potassium (18% DV), 232 mg calcium (23% DV), 101 mg magnesium (25% DV), 0.014 mcg B12 (0% DV), 0.45 mg B6 (21% DV), 4.5 mg iron (25% DV)

# Savory Spinach and Cheese "Scuffins" (Scone-Muffins!)

Craving carbs? Well then, a savory scone-muffin hybrid probably sounds pretty good to you. The downside to nausea-related carb cravings is that all those carbs can mean too little protein and veggies. And depending on your carb choices, likely too little fiber. These "scuffins" put the smack down on carb cravings while offering up protein, fiber, and veggies. And they pair SO well with soup.

---

makes 8 servings / prep time: 10 minutes / total time: 55 minutes

---

Cooking spray

3 cups old-fashioned rolled oats

2 teaspoons baking powder

1 teaspoon garlic powder

½ teaspoon baking soda

½ teaspoon smoked paprika

¼ teaspoon coarse sea salt

¾ cup 0% plain Greek yogurt

¼ cup olive oil

¼ cup skim milk or unsweetened dairy-free alternative

1 large egg, lightly beaten

1 (15-ounce) can chickpeas, rinsed and drained

¾ cup shredded cheddar cheese

4 cups baby spinach, chopped

Preheat the oven to 350°F. Coat a large muffin tin with cooking spray.

Blend the oats in a blender until they turn into a powder, about 45 seconds, stopping to stir if they get packed at the bottom of the blender. Pour the oat mixture into a large bowl. Stir in the baking powder, garlic powder, baking soda, paprika, and salt and set aside. In a separate bowl, whisk together the yogurt, oil, milk, and egg, then stir into the oat mixture until fully incorporated and no lumps remain. Stir in the chickpeas and cheese. Stir in the spinach, one cup at a time, pushing it into the mixture until all 4 cups are incorporated. You might want to use your hands for this, which makes it a bit easier to squish the spinach into the dough.

Form the dough into 8 rounds and place each into the wells of the muffin tin. Bake until firm and golden on top, about 45 minutes.

Per serving: 291 calories, 13 g protein, 30 g carbohydrates, 7 g fiber, 2 g total sugar, 14 g fat, 4 g saturated fat, 373 mg sodium, 298 mg potassium (9% DV), 215 mg calcium (22% DV), 69 mg magnesium (17% DV), 0.357 mcg B12 (6% DV), 0.102 mg B6 (5% DV), 2.4 mg iron (13% DV)

Healthy, Happy Pregnancy Cookbook

# Carrot-Ginger Soup

Sometimes a meal of soup is the only thing you can stomach. But it can be difficult to find soups that aren't packed with meat (and the accompanying meaty smell) that still deliver enough protein. Bone broth is the key to a soup that packs in protein, but stays smooth. A cup of bone broth delivers 9 grams of protein, compared to regular broth's 1 gram of protein per cup. This soup has a fresh, light flavor without a heavy scent and it manages to deliver major nutrition benefits, including 20 grams of protein per serving, anti-nausea ginger, and B vitamins. It's also delicious and easy to freeze or tote with you as a work lunch.

makes 4 servings (2 cups each) / prep time: 5 minutes / total time: 55 minutes

**2 tablespoons olive oil**

**2 pounds carrots (about 10 large), sliced into ¼-inch coins**

**1 large yellow onion, chopped**

**4 cups chicken bone broth (Pacific organic brand is in many grocery stores)**

**1 (15-ounce) can white beans, rinsed and drained**

**1 cup water**

**1½ tablespoons chopped fresh ginger**

**½ teaspoon salt**

In a large saucepan, heat the oil over medium heat. Add the carrots and onion and cook, covered, until the onion is tender but not brown, about 15 minutes. Add the broth, beans, water, ginger, and salt. Simmer, covered, until the carrots are soft, about 30 minutes more.

Using an immersion blender, puree the mixture until smooth. Or, if you prefer a chunkier soup, puree only until you reach a texture you love. You can also blend in smaller batches using a regular blender.

Per serving: 335 calories, 20 g protein, 50 g carbohydrates, 13 g fiber, 13 g total sugar, 8 g fat, 1 g saturated fat, 584 mg sodium, 1310 mg potassium (37% DV), 168 mg calcium (17% DV), 90 mg magnesium (23% DV), 0 mcg B12 (0% DV), 0.448 mg B6 (22% DV), 4.2 mg iron (24% DV)

# Orange and Pumpkin Seed Spinach Salad

This salad delivers a hearty boost of protein, without having to fill your kitchen with the scents of cooking protein that used to be appealing to you but now make you want to hurl. In addition, the orange adds a bright flavor and a slight tartness that many women report helps to ease "the queasies." The protein and abundant B vitamins can also help tame that queasy feeling.

makes 4 servings / prep time: 10 minutes / total time: 10 minutes

⅔ cup shelled raw pumpkin seeds, divided

3 tablespoons olive oil

3 tablespoons champagne vinegar or apple cider vinegar

2½ tablespoons minced shallots

1 teaspoon Dijon mustard

½ teaspoon coarse sea salt

⅛ teaspoon freshly ground black pepper

¼ teaspoon ground coriander

4 cups baby spinach

1½ cups diced unpeeled English cucumbers (¼-inch pieces)

2 large oranges, peeled and chopped (½-inch chunks), divided

1 (15-ounce) can white beans, rinsed and drained, divided

In a small skillet, toast the pumpkin seeds over medium heat, stirring constantly, until they begin to brown and emit a toasted smell, about 3 minutes. Set aside. Whisk together the oil, vinegar, shallots, mustard, salt, pepper, and coriander and set aside.

In a large salad bowl, toss the spinach and cucumber with half of the dressing, half the chopped oranges, half the pumpkin seeds, and half the beans. Top with the remaining beans and orange chunks. Drizzle the remaining half of the dressing over the top. Finish by sprinkling on the remainder of the pumpkin seeds. Toss again gently.

Per serving: 397 calories, 16 g protein, 42 g carbohydrates, 10 g fiber, 11 g total sugar, 20 g fat, 3 g saturated fat, 190 mg sodium, 1113 mg potassium (32% DV), 173 mg calcium (17% DV), 208 mg magnesium (52% DV), 0 mcg B12 (0% DV), 0.269 mg B6 (13% DV), 6.2 mg iron (35% DV)

# Cod en Papillote with Lemon-Balsamic Fennel

If you're craving fish for dinner but the thought of smelling cooking fish makes you gag (hey, pregnancy nausea is a fickle creature) then cooking en papillote is for you. Because the fish is cooked enclosed in parchment wrappers, you get less fish smell filling your kitchen. This cooking method also cooks your veggies at the same time and adds major flavor to food while being so low maintenance. Partner this cod with whatever carbohydrate option is sounding best to you at the moment—we love it with quinoa or brown rice.

makes 4 servings / prep time: 5 minutes / total time: 25 minutes

---

**4 (4-ounce) cod fillets**

**1 teaspoon lemon zest**

**Juice of ½ lemon**

**2 tablespoons balsamic vinegar**

**2 tablespoons olive oil**

**½ teaspoon coarse sea salt**

**1 cup fresh flat-leaf parsley, finely chopped**

**½ medium yellow onion, thinly sliced**

**1 medium fennel bulb, trimmed and thinly sliced**

Preheat the oven to 400°F. Place a piece of cod in the center of each of 4 large pieces of parchment paper or aluminum foil.

Whisk the lemon zest and juice with the vinegar, oil, salt, and parsley. Place one-quarter of the onion slices onto each piece of fish, followed by one-quarter of the fennel. Drizzle one-quarter of the vinegar mixture over each piece of fish, then fold the parchment paper in half around the fish and crimp the edges until you've formed a tightly sealed packet around each fillet.

Bake the packets on a baking sheet until the fish is firm and the parchment paper is starting to get crispy and brown, about 18 minutes.

Per serving: 172 calories, 21 g protein, 6 g carbohydrates, 2 g fiber, 3 g total sugar, 7 g fat, 1 g saturated fat, 322 mg sodium, 651 mg potassium (19% DV), 78 mg calcium (8% DV), 49 mg magnesium (12% DV), 0 mcg B12 (0% DV), 0.082 mg B6 (4% DV), 1.4 mg iron (8% DV)

# Cashew–Pinto Bean Burgers

These patties have it all—fiber, protein, healthy fat, crunchy texture, soft texture, delicious flavor. They can also be made ahead and frozen and reheated for a quick meal. Their protein and B vitamins can help combat nausea, and the fact that they don't have a strong smell and they pair well with any food (toss one on a salad, put an egg or sautéed tofu on top, chop up and add to pasta, top with avocado or marinara and mozzarella, etc.) makes them a versatile player in your mealtime toolbox.

makes 4 servings (four 4-inch patties) / prep time: 10 minutes / total time: 20 minutes

1 cup diced eggplant

4 teaspoons olive oil, divided

1 (15-ounce) can pinto beans, rinsed and drained, divided

½ cup whole cashews, divided

1 teaspoon chili powder

½ teaspoon ground cumin

½ teaspoon garlic powder

½ teaspoon coarse sea salt

3 tablespoons water

1 cup cooked buckwheat

In a skillet, sauté the eggplant in 2 teaspoons of the oil over medium-high heat until golden, about 5 minutes. In a blender or food processor, blend half the beans with half the cashews, the chili powder, cumin, garlic, salt, and water until smooth, about 1 minute. Coarsely chop the remaining half of the cashews and stir into the blended mixture, along with the eggplant, the remaining whole beans, and the buckwheat. Form into 4-inch-wide patties.

Heat the remaining 2 teaspoons oil in the skillet over medium heat and cook the burgers until golden on both sides, about 5 minutes per side.

Per serving: 270 calories, 11 g protein, 31 g carbohydrates, 7 g fiber, 3 g total sugar, 14 g fat, 2 g saturated fat, 416 mg sodium, 354 mg potassium (10% DV), 63 mg calcium (6% DV), 90 mg magnesium (23% DV), 0 mcg B12 (0% DV), 0.191 mg B6 (10% DV), 2.6 mg iron (14% DV)

# Lemon-Ginger Zing Cubes

These cubes are not for the faint of heart . . . but they are for the nauseated. A strong (emphasis on strong) ginger flavor dominates and helps soothe an upset stomach, while the tart lemon delivers a bright flavor. Pop one first thing in the morning or whenever nausea strikes. Or plop one or two into a glass of seltzer water for a sort of homemade lemon-ginger ale.

makes 16 servings (1 cube per serving) / prep time: 5 minutes / total time: 5 minutes + overnight freezing

**¾ cup freshly squeezed lemon juice (about 5 large lemons)**

**¾ cup water**

**¼ cup honey**

**2 tablespoons grated fresh ginger**

Puree the lemon juice, water, honey, and ginger in a blender until smooth, about 1 minute. Strain through a fine-mesh sieve or cheesecloth into an ice-cube tray and freeze until solid, 4 hours or overnight.

Per serving: 20 calories, 0 g protein, 5 g carbohydrates, 0 g fiber, 5 g total sugar, 0 g fat, 0 g saturated fat, 0 mg sodium, 20 mg potassium (.6% DV), 1 mg calcium (0% DV), 1 mg magnesium (0% DV), 0 mcg B12 (0% DV), 0.008 mg B6 (0% DV), 0 mg iron (0% DV)

# Hemp-Coconut Oatmeal Cookie Energy Bites

Going too long without eating can trigger nausea, but having a nutritionally balanced snack on hand isn't always a simple task. Until now! These energy bites can be stashed in a bag and taken to work or on an errand-run so when hunger hits, you've got an answer. And before you roll your eyes about the chopped raisins . . . there's a method to our madness. These bites don't have any added sweetener—the only sweetness comes from the raisins. This is rare and made possible by the fact that the raisins are chopped into small pieces so the sweetness is more evenly dispersed into each bite.

makes 6 servings (1 bite per serving) / prep time: 5 minutes / total time: 5 minutes + 1 hour refrigeration

⅓ cup old-fashioned rolled oats

½ cup raisins, packed, finely chopped

3 tablespoons unsweetened shredded coconut

2 tablespoons hemp seeds

1 teaspoon ground cinnamon

¼ teaspoon ground ginger

Pinch of nutmeg

⅓ cup salted natural almond butter

Stir the oats, raisins, coconut, hemp seeds, cinnamon, ginger, and nutmeg in a medium bowl until all the ingredients are thoroughly combined.

Add the almond butter, pressing it into the oat mixture with a spatula or spoon until evenly dispersed. Press and knead the mixture with your hands until all of the ingredients are mixed together and form a large ball. Divide into 6 pieces, rolling each piece into a small ball. Refrigerate for at least 1 hour before eating to allow flavors to meld. Energy bites can be refrigerated for up to 2 weeks.

Per serving: 180 calories, 5 g protein, 18 g carbohydrates, 3 g fiber, 9 g total sugar, 11 g fat, 2.5 g saturated fat, 34 mg sodium, 239 mg potassium (7% DV), 65 mg calcium (7% DV), 72 mg magnesium (18% DV), 0 mcg B12 (0% DV), 0.069 mg B6 (3% DV), 1.5 mg iron (8.5% DV)

# CHAPTER TWO

# I Have "Cankles": Recipes to Ease Water Retention

Oh hormones! You nutty things! It seems like each chapter in this book is the result, at least in part, of the symptoms from hormonal changes. Fluid retention is no exception. Increased hormones during pregnancy cause your body to hold onto more fluid—your blood/fluid volume increases about 50 percent during pregnancy. This is a good thing, since you need more blood and fluid to support a healthy pregnancy. The swollen feet and ankles you see (or don't see, depending on your growing bump) are most often caused by gravity as well as pressure from the baby on blood vessels in your abdomen that can slow the flow of blood from your lower limbs up. Warm weather, dehydration, and salty foods are other common causes of increased fluid retention.

Staying hydrated is one of the most important ways to minimize fluid retention. Reducing salt intake, so it doesn't go above daily recommendations (no more than 2400 mg daily), in addition to including potassium-rich foods on the regular (they help flush out excess sodium) is extremely helpful. And since many fruits and veggies are loaded with potassium, naturally low in sodium, and packed with water, they will become your new best friends.

# Smart Sips: Herb Waters

Add any of the following combinations to 64 ounces of fresh, filtered water and let sit for at least 2 hours before enjoying. Once that water is gone, you can refill with plain water one more time to enjoy a second batch of flavored water.

## Cinnamon-Orange

**1 cinnamon stick, broken into pieces**
**4 slices unpeeled orange**

## Cucumber-Mint

**6 slices fresh unpeeled cucumber**
**4 sprigs fresh mint**

## Rosemary-Lemon

**1 sprig fresh rosemary, lightly rolled between hands to bruise leaves**
**4 slices unpeeled lemon**

Healthy, Happy Pregnancy Cookbook

# Carrot Cake Chia Pudding

     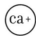

If you haven't had chia pudding yet, then you're reading the right recipe because this dish combines the creaminess of chia pudding with the flavors of carrot cake. Win-win. Chia seeds (ch- ch- ch- chia!) can absorb up to ten times their weight in water, which means that when you eat the soaked seeds they release that water for your hydration benefit.

makes 4 servings / prep time: 15 minutes / total time: 15 minutes + overnight

1 teaspoon coconut oil

2 carrots, shredded

1 tablespoon ground cinnamon

3½ cups skim milk or unsweetened dairy-free alternative

1 banana

¼ cup plus 2 tablespoons raisins

1 teaspoon pure vanilla extract

½ cup plus 2 tablespoons chia seeds

Cashew Cream

¼ cup cashews

1 cup water, plus 2 tablespoons

¼ teaspoon pure vanilla extract

½ teaspoon honey

Dash of ground cinnamon

Heat the oil in a medium skillet over medium heat. Toss the carrots with the cinnamon and cook in the oil for 5 minutes until they are beginning to soften but not at all brown. Set aside and let the carrots cool completely.

Add the cooled carrots to a blender with the milk, banana, raisins, and vanilla. Blend on high until fully pureed. Transfer to a bowl. Stir in the chia seeds and store in the refrigerator for 4 hours or overnight before eating.

To make the cashew cream, soak the cashews in the 1 cup of water for at least 3 hours. Drain and add to a small blender or food processor with the 2 tablespoons water, vanilla, honey, and cinnamon. Blend until smooth. Top each serving of chia pudding with a spoonful of cashew cream.

Per serving: 391 calories, 16 g protein, 51 g carbohydrates, 16 g fiber, 25 g total sugar, 16 g fat, 3 g saturated fat, 120 mg sodium, 841 mg potassium (24% DV), 533 mg calcium (53% DV), 182 mg magnesium (46% DV), 1.136 mcg B12 (19% DV), 0.524 mg B6 (26% DV), 3.9 mg iron (22% DV)

# Potato Benedict

Potatoes deserve a lot more praise than they get. They've got more water retention–busting potassium than bananas, contain a special type of fiber called resistant starch that can help feed your good gut bacteria, and are so super delicious that they make your taste buds sing. Spuds are also really versatile, and they're a great way to replace more refined carbohydrates with a higher fiber, less refined carb source. This recipe skips the typical English muffin and uses flattened potatoes as the throne for the eggs and sauce.

makes 2 servings / prep time: 5 minutes / total time: 15 minutes

2 medium red or purple potatoes

1 tablespoon plus 1 teaspoon olive oil

2 pinches coarse sea salt

¼ cup low-fat plain Greek yogurt

1¼ teaspoons mustard (grainy, Dijon, or yellow)

½ teaspoon dried dill

½ teaspoon freshly squeezed lemon juice

2 thick tomato slices

4 large eggs, poached (see Six Easy Ways to Cook Eggs, page 29)

2 tablespoons finely chopped fresh flat-leaf parsley

Poke a fork into each potato in three or four places and microwave on high until they begin to soften, about 4 minutes. Flip over and microwave on high until soft all the way through, an additional 3 minutes.

Slice each potato in half lengthwise and allow to cool slightly. Using the bottom of a mug, gently press each potato half to flatten it slightly. Sauté the potato halves in the oil over medium-high heat until browned on both sides, about 3 minutes total. Sprinkle lightly with a pinch of salt.

Whisk together the yogurt, mustard, dill, lemon juice, and remaining pinch of salt. Top each potato half with a slice of tomato, a poached egg, and half of the yogurt mixture. Sprinkle with the parsley and serve.

Per serving: 402 calories, 20 g protein, 38 g carbohydrates, 4 g fiber, 5 g total sugar, 19 g fat, 5 g saturated fat, 287 mg sodium, 1204 mg potassium (34% DV), 120 mg calcium (12% DV), 67 mg magnesium (17% DV), 1.29 mcg B12 (22% DV), 0.538 mg B6 (27% DV), 4 mg iron (22% DV)

# Banana Bread–Yogurt Parfait

This parfait of deliciousness is truly fast food. But unlike the fast food you pick up from a drive-thru, this meal was made with love, using fresh ingredients in your very own kitchen. It's also a home run when you're making breakfast for a group, such as unexpected out-of-town guests or your prenatal yoga friends. The combination of mega potassium, very little sodium, and watery foods (fruit and yogurt both contain lots of water) makes this dish a serious puff-fighter. Plus, if you make it the night before in individual glass jars, you can officially be one of those super-pulled-together people who eat breakfast out of a cute jar. Just don't forget to document it with a picture.

makes 4 servings / prep time: 5 minutes / total time: 5 minutes

---

3 bananas, divided

4 cups low-fat plain yogurt

2 teaspoons pure vanilla extract

2 teaspoons ground cinnamon, divided

1 cup old-fashioned rolled oats, divided

½ cup chopped walnuts

In a medium bowl, mash 2 of the bananas. Stir in the yogurt, vanilla, 1 teaspoon of the cinnamon, and ½ cup of the oats.

Slice the remaining banana and toss with the remaining 1 teaspoon cinnamon, remaining ½ cup oats, and the walnuts.

Place ½ cup of the yogurt mixture into each of four tall, narrow glasses or jars. Top each with ¼ cup of the banana-walnut mixture. Divide the remaining yogurt mixture evenly on top of the banana-walnut layer in each glass and then finish by topping each with one-quarter of the remaining banana-walnut mixture.

*Note:* The parfaits can be made the night before and stored in the fridge or even kept in the fridge for several days if you want to prep ahead for the end of the week!

Per serving: 429 calories, 19 g protein, 58 g carbohydrates, 6 g fiber, 31 g total sugar, 15 g fat, 3.5 g saturated fat, 174 mg sodium, 1087 mg potassium (31% DV), 492 mg calcium (49% DV), 122 mg magnesium (31% DV), 1.372 mcg B12 (23% DV), 0.598 mg B6 (30% DV), 1.9 mg iron (10% DV)

# Fiesta Bowl Salad with Cilantro-Lime Dressing

This salad is silly-fast to make. It's also silly-delicious, great as leftovers, and makes a fantastic dip for corn chips. The flavors will satisfy any Mexican food cravings, but with a much lower sodium level (and much higher fiber level) than ordering out. So, your taste buds, your ankles, and your schedule will thank you.

makes 4 servings / prep time: 10 minutes / total time: 10 minutes

**2 bell peppers, diced**

**2 cups cooked fresh corn kernals, or frozen and thawed**

**2 (15-ounce) cans black beans, rinsed and drained**

**1 large tomato, diced**

**1 avocado, diced**

**1 cup fresh cilantro leaves**

**1 teaspoon grated lime zest**

**3 tablespoons freshly squeezed lime juice**

**¼ cup olive oil**

**1 teaspoon honey**

**½ teaspoon coarse sea salt**

**¼ teaspoon freshly ground black pepper**

**¼ teaspoon ground coriander**

**½ teaspoon ground cumin**

Combine the bell peppers, corn, beans, tomato, and avocado in a large bowl.

In a small food processor or blender, puree the cilantro, lime zest, lime juice, oil, honey, salt, black pepper, coriander, and cumin, until smooth. Pour the dressing over the corn mixture and gently toss to coat.

Per serving: 438 calories, 15 g protein, 56 g carbohydrates, 19 g fiber, 10 g total sugar, 20 g fat, 3.0 g saturated fat, 287 mg sodium, 762 mg potassium (22% DV), 33 mg calcium (3% DV), 58 mg magnesium (15% DV), 0 mcg B12 (0% DV), 0.396 mg B6 (20% DV), 16 mg iron (90% DV)

# Crunchy Salmon Salad Wrap

Crunchy salmon rolls are a sushi dinner favorite, and this recipe combines the best of those rolls (crunchy texture, delicious salmon, and great flavor) with something you can make at home and safely eat while pregnant. Plus, these wraps have a lot less sodium and a whole lot more potassium and fiber than soy sauce–dunked sushi rolls.

makes 2 servings / prep time: 10 minutes / total time: 10 minutes

1 (5-ounce) can boneless, skinless wild salmon, drained and flaked

¼ cup chopped red onion

1 large carrot, chopped

1 celery stalk, chopped

¼ cup roasted unsalted sunflower seeds, shelled

1½ tablespoons mayonnaise

1½ teaspoons Dijon mustard

½ teaspoon dried dill

Scant ¼ teaspoon sea salt

¼ teaspoon garlic powder

¼ teaspoon chili powder

⅛ teaspoon freshly ground black pepper

1½ tablespoons apple cider vinegar

2 small nori/seaweed sheets, crumbled

2 (10-inch) whole grain tortillas

In a medium bowl, mix the salmon, onion, carrot, celery, and sunflower seeds. In a separate bowl, whisk together the mayo, mustard, dill, salt, garlic powder, chili powder, pepper, and vinegar until smooth.

Pour the dressing over the salmon mixture and stir until evenly coated. Stir in the nori sheets. Place half the salmon mixture in the center of each of the tortillas and roll up.

Per serving: 420 calories, 21 g protein, 41 g carbohydrates, 8 g fiber, 4 g total sugar, 21 g fat, 3.0 g saturated fat, 663 mg sodium, 614 mg potassium (19% DV), 82 mg calcium (8% DV), 76 mg magnesium (19% DV), 0.034 mcg B12 (0% DV), 0.396 mg B6 (20% DV), 3.1 mg iron (17% DV)

# Chili-Stuffed Delicata Squash

What's cooler than a bread bowl? An edible squash bowl filled with chili. Plus, starchy squashes, such as delicata, provide fiber, vitamin power, and major potassium—and they don't get soggy at the end of the meal. And you can eat them as leftovers without them turning to a paste. Wow! Bread bowls aren't sounding that cool anymore. Squash bowls are where it's at!

---

makes 4 servings / prep time: 15 minutes / total time: 1 hour

---

Olive oil spray

2 large delicata squash (or acorn squash if you can't find delicata)

¾ teaspoon sea salt, divided

1 tablespoon extra-virgin olive oil

1 cup chopped red or yellow onion

2 garlic cloves, minced

1 pound ground grass-fed beef or bison

1 tablespoon chili powder

2 tablespoons tomato paste

2 teaspoons dried oregano

2 teaspoons ground cumin

½ teaspoon ground cinnamon

¼ teaspoon freshly ground black pepper

2 tablespoons finely chopped seeded poblano peppers, or 1 (4-ounce) can mild green chiles (optional—use only if you like spicy foods)

1 (15-ounce) can kidney beans, rinsed and drained

1 (14.5-ounce) can diced tomatoes, with their juice

Preheat the oven to 400°F. Coat a baking sheet with olive oil spray.

Cut both squash in half lengthwise and discard the seeds. Place the squash halves facedown on the baking sheet and bake until softened, 25 to 30 minutes. Remove from the oven, flip the halves over, and season with ½ teaspoon of the salt, sprinkling it evenly over the 4 halves.

While the squash cooks, heat the oil in large saucepan over medium heat. Add the onion and garlic. Sauté until the onion softens, about 5 minutes. Add the meat and cook, breaking the meat up with a wooden spoon, until crumbled and browned, about 10 minutes more. Stir in all the remaining ingredients (chili powder through tomatoes) and the remaining ¼ teaspoon salt and bring to a boil. Reduce the heat and simmer until the mixture has thickened and most of the liquid has evaporated, about 22 minutes.

Fill each squash half with one-quarter of the chili mixture. Bake the squash until fork-tender, about 10 minutes more.

Per serving: 438 calories, 34 g protein, 53 g carbohydrates, 13 g fiber, 12 g total sugar, 13 g fat, 4.0 g saturated fat, 532 mg sodium, 2052 mg potassium (59% DV), 160 mg calcium (16% DV), 108 mg magnesium (27% DV), 2.2 mcg B12 (37% DV), 1.111 mg B6 (56% DV), 7.7 mg iron (43% DV)

# (Better Than) Fried Mushrooms

If you like biting into a crunchy, flavorful coating to find a perfectly cooked mushroom, you are going to love this recipe. And these tasty bites are more than just a pretty face; they've got nutritional substance, too. These babies pack in potassium while adding major flavor with spices so you can get away with using a lot less salt than restaurant-style breaded mushrooms.

makes 2 servings / prep time: 15 minutes / total time: 40 minutes

Olive oil spray

1 large egg

2 teaspoons water

1 teaspoon chili powder, divided

1 teaspoon garlic powder, divided

½ teaspoon ground turmeric, divided

½ teaspoon smoked paprika, divided

¼ teaspoon sea salt, plus a pinch

¼ teaspoon freshly ground black pepper, divided

½ cup plain bread crumbs

14 cremini mushrooms, stems removed

Preheat the oven to 425°F. Coat a baking sheet with olive oil spray.

In a small bowl, whisk the egg with the water, ½ teaspoon of the chili powder, ½ teaspoon of the garlic powder, ¼ teaspoon of the turmeric, ¼ teaspoon of the smoked paprika, a pinch of salt, and ⅛ teaspoon of the pepper.

In a small dish, stir the bread crumbs with the remaining ½ teaspoon chili powder, ½ teaspoon garlic powder, ¼ teaspoon turmeric, ¼ teaspoon smoked paprika, the ¼ teaspoon salt, and the remaining ⅛ teaspoon pepper.

Dip each mushroom into the egg mixture to fully coat. Shake off excess egg and gently coat the mushroom in the bread crumbs. Once the mushrooms are coated, working with one mushroom at a time, quickly dip the coated mushrooms back into egg mixture and coat once again in bread crumbs. Place the bread crumb–covered mushrooms, cap side up, on the baking sheet. Lightly spray the tops with more olive oil.

Bake until the mushrooms are golden brown and crispy, about 25 minutes, turning halfway through the baking time.

Per serving: 167 calories, 10 g protein, 22 g carbohydrates, 3 g fiber, 5 g total sugar, 5 g fat, 1.0 g saturated fat, 349 mg sodium, 661 mg potassium (19% DV), 84 mg calcium (8% DV), 16 mg magnesium (4% DV), 0.462 mcg B12 (8% DV), 0.19 mg B6 (10% DV), 2.1 mg iron (12% DV)

# Homemade Green "Juice"

If a smoothie and juice had a baby, this drink would be it. Unlike juices made in juicers, this one retains all of the fiber and nutrients since you're sipping the whole veggies and fruit, skin and all. In addition, you're hydrating at the same time you're getting potassium, a combination that acts as the mortal enemy of fluid retention.

makes 2 servings / prep time: 1 minute / total time: 4 minutes

**2 apples, chopped**

**2 cups coarsely chopped kale**

**2 cups water**

**1½ cups chopped cucumbers
(preferably organic and unpeeled)**

**1 large celery stalk, chopped**

**⅓ cup chopped fresh curly-leaf
parsley**

**1 tablespoon freshly squeezed
lemon juice**

Place the apples, kale, water, cucumber, celery, parsley, and lemon juice in the blender and blend on high until smooth, about 3 minutes. Drink immediately. If you prefer a less pulpy juice, pour through a mesh sieve while gently pushing through with a spoon.

Per serving: 126 calories, 4 g protein, 29 g carbohydrates, 6 g fiber, 16 g total sugar, 1 g fat, 0 g saturated fat, 60 mg sodium, 746 mg potassium (21% DV), 148 mg calcium (15% DV), 58 mg magnesium (15% DV), 0 mcg B12 (0% DV), 0.32 mg B6 (16% DV), 2 mg iron (11% DV)

# the dirty dozen PLUS

Some plants get more pesticides during growing and some produce naturally catches and traps pesticides, while others aren't exposed to as many pesticides or don't retain much of the ones they are exposed to. For instance, peaches have a fuzzy skin that holds onto pesticides like Leo held Kate in *Titanic*. The same goes for strawberries, with their teeny nooks and crannies. The kind folks at the Environmental Working Group (www.EWG.org) tested pesticide residue on produce and created a list of the twelve most pesticide-laden fruits and veggies. These are best purchased organic to reduce your (and baby's) exposure to pesticides. They also added two that contain trace levels of highly hazardous pesticides and should be purchased organic if you eat them often. And if you can't find an organic version, skip them in lieu of something not on the list.

1. Apples
2. Celery
3. Cherry tomatoes
4. Cucumbers
5. Grapes
6. Nectarines
7. Peaches
8. Potatoes
9. Snap peas
10. Spinach
11. Strawberries
12. Sweet bell peppers
PLUS Hot peppers
PLUS Kale/Collard greens

# should you choose organic?

The benefits of opting for organic food as often as possible are far-reaching: less pesticide exposure for you, baby, and Mother Nature. The downside is that organic options can be more expensive and, depending on your location, harder to find. Shop seasonally, watch the sales at your local grocery stores, and visit local farmers' markets whenever possible. Choose the organic version of foods as often as you can. However, if you're making the choice between eating conventionally grown produce or not eating produce at all, by all means choose the conventional produce and wash it well. Any fruits and veggies are better than no fruits and veggies. And remember that when it comes to packaged foods (cereal, chips, crackers, cookies, etc.), being organic does not automatically mean it's a healthy choice. Scour that ingredient list no matter what.

# Raspberry Swirl Frozen Yogurt Pops

These pops pack a major potassium punch. Try saying that five times fast! Not only does the potassium in these pops help reduce fluid retention, but your taste buds will be doing a happy dance, too. And, as if you needed another benefit to these tasty treats, you get a fruit and fiber boost with each one!

makes 4 servings / prep time: 10 minutes + 30 minutes soaking time / total time: 10 minutes + overnight freezing

**4 Medjool or Deglet Noor dates, pitted**

**2 tablespoons water, plus more for soaking**

**1 cup frozen and thawed raspberries**

**¾ cup full-fat plain Greek yogurt or dairy-free alternative**

Soak the dates in warm water until soft, at least 30 minutes. Puree the raspberries and water in a blender until smooth, about 1 minute. Add 2 dates and blend again until the dates are completely pureed, about 2 minutes more. Pour the mixture into a glass and set aside.

Add the yogurt and remaining 2 dates to a clean blender container and blend on high until the dates are pureed, about 2 minutes.

In each of 4 ice pop molds (or 6 molds if they're smaller), layer 2 large spoonfuls of the yogurt followed by 2 spoonfuls of the raspberry puree. Repeat until all of the yogurt and raspberry puree are used. Slide a butter knife down the insides of the molds to swirl the mixtures.

Freeze the pops overnight.

Per serving: 123 calories, 5 g protein, 23 g carbohydrates, 4 g fiber, 17 g total sugar, 2 g fat, 1 g saturated fat, 20 mg sodium, 214 mg potassium (6% DV), 49 mg calcium (5% DV), 20 mg magnesium (5% DV), 0 mcg B12 (0% DV), 0.077 mg B6 (4% DV), 0.4 mg iron (2% DV)

# CHAPTER THREE

# My Chest is On Fire: Recipes to Prevent Heartburn

Just when the nausea of the first trimester goes away, heartburn often appears. Is your body trying to torture you? Please don't take it personally; there are several reasons you might develop heartburn in your second and third trimester. Your body having a personal vendetta against you is not one of them. Pregnancy hormones are. Certain hormones that increase during pregnancy cause muscle relaxation, including the muscle that controls the valve between your stomach and your esophagus. So, it's more likely that acid from your stomach can work its way up into your throat and cause that burning sensation. Also, as your growing baby takes up more of your abdominal real estate, organs get pushed around and your stomach gets crowded. This can cause the stomach contents (including acid) to be pushed upward toward your esophagus.

The good news is that there are certain foods that tend to trigger heartburn more than others. That is good news because once you know which foods are triggers, you can avoid them. And it's even better news because this entire chapter has delicious, satisfying, and good-for-you recipes that shun all the major triggers: chocolate, tomato, mint, citrus, coffee/tea, spicy foods, onion, garlic, black pepper.

# Cauliflower and Cheddar Omelet

Mirepoix is a fancy way of saying chopped onion, celery, and carrots that you can use as the base of nearly any savory dish to make it taste totally awesome. This omelet has a mirepoix that is lacking in onion (so you skip the heartburn) but not in rich, savory flavor. It's also loaded with protein, to keep you extra-satisfied without feeling overly stuffed.

makes 2 servings / prep time: 5 minutes / total time: 25 minutes

4 teaspoons olive oil, divided

2 tablespoons finely chopped celery

2 tablespoons finely chopped carrots

1 cup finely chopped cauliflower

Pinch of coarse sea salt

4 large eggs

1 tablespoon water

½ teaspoon dried oregano

½ cup shredded cheddar cheese

In a medium skillet, heat 2 teaspoons of the oil over medium heat. Add the celery and carrots and sauté until they begin to soften, about 4 minutes. Add the cauliflower and salt and continue to cook, stirring often, until the cauliflower is soft and lightly browned, about 8 minutes more. Set aside the veggie mixture and lightly wipe out the skillet with a paper towel.

In a bowl, whisk the eggs, water, and oregano. Heat the remaining 2 teaspoons oil in the skillet over medium heat. Add the egg mixture and, using a spatula, gently push through the egg mixture a couple times as it begins to cook so the liquid egg at the top makes contact with the pan's surface. Cook the eggs until just firm, about 3½ minutes. Sprinkle the veggie mixture and the cheese onto half of the cooked omelet and fold the empty side over the filling to cover. Cook until the cheese has melted, about 2 minutes more.

Per serving: 354 calories, 21 g protein, 5 g carbohydrates, 2 g fiber, 3 g total sugar, 28 g fat, 10.5 g saturated fat, 356 mg sodium, 362 mg potassium (10% DV), 277 mg calcium (28% DV), 30 mg magnesium (8% DV), 1.524 mcg B12 (25% DV), 0.294 mg B6 (15% DV), 2.4 mg iron (13% DV)

Healthy, Happy Pregnancy Cookbook

# Pistachio-Cardamom Baked Apple with Vanilla Cream

You know when you drink really tasty chai tea and you think, "What is that flavor?" The answer is cardamom. It tastes like perfume, but in a good way, similar to jasmine tea's "perfume-y" quality. Paired with the sweetness of baked apple and the warm flavor of vanilla, along with 7 grams of fiber per serving, these baked apples satisfy on every level.

makes 4 servings / prep time: 10 minutes / total time: 1 hour

4 large apples

¼ cup water

½ cup chopped pistachios, divided

½ teaspoon ground cardamom, divided

7 teaspoons honey, divided

4 teaspoons salted butter, divided

2 cups low-fat plain Greek yogurt

2 teaspoons pure vanilla extract

Preheat the oven to 375°F. Using a paring knife, begin cutting out the stem and upper core of the apple, but leave the lower quarter of the core intact. This way, what you stuff into the apple won't fall out. Place the apples in a baking dish with about ¼ cup of water on the bottom.

Place 1 tablespoon of the pistachios into the center of each apple and top each with ⅛ teaspoon of the cardamom and 1 teaspoon of the honey.

Place 1 teaspoon of the butter on top of the pistachio stuffing in each apple, cover with aluminum foil, and bake for 30 minutes. Remove the foil and bake, uncovered, for an additional 10 minutes.

Whisk the yogurt with the remaining 3 teaspoons honey and the vanilla. Top each baked apple with one-quarter of the yogurt mixture (about ½ cup) and 1 tablespoon of the remaining chopped pistachios.

Per serving: 360 calories, 14 g protein, 49 g carbohydrates, 7 g fiber, 37 g total sugar, 11 g fat, 5.0 g saturated fat, 81 mg sodium, 395 mg potassium (12% DV), 157 mg calcium (16% DV), 29 mg magnesium (7% DV), 0.008 mcg B12 (0% DV), 0.264 mg B6 (13% DV), 1.5 mg iron (8% DV)

# Cinnamon Breakfast Polenta with Sautéed Pears

    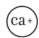

A bowl of hot cereal is one of the most soothing morning breakfast rituals around. This one combines cinnamon and sautéed fruit to make the whole thing taste like pie. Pie AND hot cereal—comfort breakfast to the max. And it's cooked with milk and topped with nuts, which means a protein boost in every bite.

makes 4 servings / prep time: 17 minutes / total time: 25 minutes

**5 cups skim milk or unsweetened dairy-free alternative**

**1 cup coarsely ground cornmeal**

**2 teaspoons ground cinnamon, divided**

**2 teaspoons pure vanilla extract**

**4 teaspoons sunflower seed oil**

**2 large ripe pears, thinly sliced**

**8 teaspoons chopped walnuts**

**2 teaspoons pure maple syrup**

Bring the milk to a boil in a large saucepan, watching carefully so it doesn't bubble over the sides of the pan. Reduce to a simmer and whisk in the cornmeal and 1 teaspoon of the cinnamon. Continue to simmer, stirring constantly, until the mixture has thickened and become smooth and creamy, about 20 minutes. Stir in the vanilla. (Note: If you choose to use quick-cooking cornmeal—also called quick-cooking polenta—the total cook time will be 5 to 10 minutes.) If you like a slightly thinner cereal consistency, add an additional ½ to 1 cup of milk or water, ¼ cup at a time, until you reach the desired consistency.

While the cornmeal cooks, heat the oil in a small skillet over medium heat. Add the pears and sauté until golden and soft, about 5 minutes. Toss the pears with the walnuts, maple syrup, and remaining 1 teaspoon cinnamon. Stir half of the pear mixture into the polenta. Divide the polenta among 4 bowls and top each with one-quarter of the remaining pear mixture.

Per serving: 366 calories, 14 g protein, 59 g carbohydrates, 6 g fiber, 28 g total sugar, 9 g fat, 1.0 g saturated fat, 141 mg sodium, 727 mg potassium (21% DV), 414 mg calcium (41% DV), 89 mg magnesium (22% DV), 1.623 mcg B12 (27% DV), 0.265 mg B6 (13% DV), 1.6 mg iron (9% DV)

# Confetti Sweet Potato Hash (#PutAnEggOnIt)

We're not saying it's fair, but sometimes when you have heartburn, you have to skip egg and potato breakfasts because they're just too heavy and "garlic-y" (and "onion-y" and "black pepper-y"). But let us right this wrong by bringing you a homemade lighter version that has way more flavor, color, and texture than anything you'll find at a diner.

makes 4 servings / prep time: 5 minutes / total time: 35 minutes

8 teaspoons olive oil, divided

2 large unpeeled sweet potatoes (about 1½ pounds), scrubbed and diced (¼-inch pieces)

1 large red bell pepper, diced (½-inch pieces)

1 large yellow bell pepper, diced (½-inch pieces)

¾ teaspoon smoked paprika

½ teaspoon coarse sea salt

¼ teaspoon ground cumin

8 large eggs

In a large skillet, heat 5 teaspoons of the oil over medium heat and sauté the potatoes until they begin to soften, about 15 minutes. Add the peppers, paprika, salt, and cumin and continue to sauté until the peppers are soft and the potatoes are golden, about another 12 minutes. Remove from the heat and divide the mixture equally among 4 plates.

Add the remaining 3 teaspoons oil to the skillet and cook the eggs in your favorite style (scrambled, over-medium, etc.). Place 2 cooked eggs on the top of each serving of potatoes.

Per serving: 330 calories, 15 g protein, 25 g carbohydrates, 4 g fiber, 8 g total sugar, 19 g fat, 4.5 g saturated fat, 316 mg sodium, 759 mg potassium (22% DV), 98 mg calcium (10% DV), 48 mg magnesium (12% DV), 1.29 mcg B12 (22% DV), 0.608 mg B6 (30% DV), 3 mg iron (17% DV)

# Peanut Butter and Grape Muffins

If you love a classic PB&J sandwich, meet the muffin version. These muffins aren't overly sweet—in fact, their only sweeteners are the banana and grapes—which makes them perfect for breakfast because you won't get a sugar rush (and then crash). And speaking of breakfast, each muffin is a perfectly balanced meal, with an ideal blend of protein, high-fiber carbs, and healthy fat. So you can literally grab-and-go.

makes 9 servings / prep time: 10 minutes / total time: 40 minutes

Cooking spray

1½ cup old-fashioned rolled oats

1½ teaspoons baking powder

½ teaspoon baking soda

½ teaspoon ground cinnamon

2 very ripe bananas

1 cup creamy unsalted natural peanut butter

⅓ cup skim milk or unsweetened dairy-free alternative

2 large eggs

2 teaspoons pure vanilla extract

1½ cups halved grapes (quarter them if they're large)

½ cup coarsely chopped roasted peanuts

Preheat the oven to 350°F. Line a muffin tin with 9 paper wrappers. Spray the wrappers well with cooking spray.

Pulse the oats in a blender or food processor until they look like flour, about 1 minute. Pour the oat flour into a large bowl and stir in the baking powder, baking soda, and cinnamon.

In a blender, combine the bananas, peanut butter, milk, eggs, and vanilla until smooth, about 45 seconds. Pour the peanut butter mixture into the oat flour mixture and stir until just combined. Gently stir in the grapes and peanuts until evenly distributed. Pour the batter into each of the wrappers. The batter will be thick so you can take it all the way to the top of each muffin cup and even a little bit above.

Bake until the muffins are golden brown and firm, about 30 minutes. Let cool completely before eating. Store leftover muffins in the fridge for up to 1 week.

Per serving: 341 calories, 13 g protein, 32 g carbohydrates, 5 g fiber, 14 g total sugar, 20 g fat, 4.0 g saturated fat, 178 mg sodium, 505 mg potassium (14% DV), 95 mg calcium (10% DV), 90 mg magnesium (23% DV), 0.191 mcg B12 (3% DV), 0.355 mg B6 (18% DV), 1.8 mg iron (10% DV)

# Mushroom, Sage, and Parmesan Baked Brown Rice

The hearty flavors of sautéed mushrooms and Parmesan cheese are balanced with the brightness of sage so that you'll never miss the onion. In fact, let's just not even mention onions, okay? This dish pairs well with a side of green veggies and a small piece of fish or chicken, or divide into 4 servings and consider it an all-in-one dinner. And it's even better heated up the next day. #LeftoversRock.

makes 6 servings / prep time: 15 minutes / total time: 1 hour 25 minutes

4 cups sliced cremini mushrooms

1 tablespoon olive oil

1 cup low-fat milk or unsweetened dairy-free alternative

2 large eggs, lightly beaten

1 teaspoon baking powder

½ teaspoon coarse sea salt

3 cups cooked brown rice

Olive oil spray

1 cup grated Parmesan cheese or dairy-free alternative

½ cup toasted pine nuts

½ tablespoon dried sage

Preheat the oven to 375°F.

In a large skillet over medium-high heat, sauté the mushrooms in the oil until tender, browned, and all the liquid has evaporated, about 10 minutes. Set aside.

In a large bowl, stir the milk, eggs, baking powder, and salt into the cooked rice until fully mixed.

Layer the mushrooms on an 8 x 8-inch baking (or 2 quart casserole) dish coated with olive oil spray. Then layer the cheese, pine nuts, sage, and rice mixture, in that order.

Bake until golden brown and firm, about 1 hour. Let sit for 10 minutes before serving.

Per serving: 337 calories, 15 g protein, 31 g carbohydrates, 3 g fiber, 4 g total sugar, 18 g fat, 4.5 g saturated fat, 479 mg sodium, 436 mg potassium (12% DV), 314 mg calcium (31% DV), 93 mg magnesium (23% DV), 0.819 mcg B12 (14% DV), 0.272 mg B6 (14% DV), 1.9 mg iron (11% DV)

# Fennel and White Bean Salad

Fennel packs a lot of flavor and, for this reason, it makes an awesome meal base when you're avoiding certain other commonly flavorful foods like garlic and onion. Fennel delivers a rich flavor when it's roasted, but the raw form is crisp, crunchy, and bright—perfect for a refreshing salad. And because the fennel really shines, the rest of the ingredients can remain pretty simple.

makes 4 servings / prep time: 5 minutes / total time: 5 minutes

1 large fennel bulb, or 2 small-medium, trimmed and thinly sliced

2 (15-ounce) cans white beans, rinsed and drained

3 tablespoons olive oil

2 tablespoons apple cider vinegar

1 tablespoon minced shallot, optional (see Note)

2 teaspoons grainy mustard

½ teaspoon coarse sea salt

½ teaspoon honey

¼ teaspoon ground cumin

⅛ teaspoon smoked paprika

Combine the fennel and beans in a large bowl.

In a small bowl, whisk the oil, vinegar, shallot (if using), mustard, salt, honey, cumin, and paprika. Drizzle over the fennel and beans and toss lightly to coat.

*Note:* You may find that shallots won't give you heartburn, even if onions do. If that's the case, go ahead and include them. If you can't eat shallots, leave them out. The dressing is great either way!

Per serving: 368 calories, 17 g protein, 52 g carbohydrates, 12 g fiber, 3 g total sugar, 11 g fat, 1.5 g saturated fat, 228 mg sodium, 1214 mg potassium (35% DV), 196 mg calcium (20% DV), 126 mg magnesium (32% DV), 0 mcg B12 (0% DV), 0.228 mg B6 (11% DV), 7.3 mg iron (41% DV)

# Tabouli-ish (aka Tomato-less Tabouli)

Lemon juice (and other citrus juices) are a major no-no if you're experiencing heartburn, but the zest can be a way to get around the symptoms without sacrificing the crisp flavor of citrus. The fresh ingredients in this salad don't need too much help to shine, so the simple yet flavorful dressing just acts to tie all of the flavors and textures together. And like many grain dishes, this one gets better as it sits in the fridge—so look forward to leftovers.

makes 4 servings / prep time: 5 minutes / total time: 5 minutes

**3 tablespoons olive oil**

**2 teaspoons finely grated lemon zest**

**½ teaspoon coarse sea salt**

**¼ teaspoon ground cumin**

**2 cups cooked bulgur wheat**

**2 cups chopped cucumbers (¼-inch dice)**

**1 (15-ounce) can chickpeas, rinsed and drained**

**1 cup chopped fresh flat-leaf parsley**

**½ cup chopped red bell peppers (¼-inch dice)**

Whisk together the oil, lemon zest, salt, and cumin in a small bowl. Combine the bulgur, cucumbers, chickpeas, parsley, and bell peppers in a large bowl. Pour the dressing over the bulgur mixture and toss well to coat all the ingredients with the dressing.

Per serving: 253 calories, 8 g protein, 31 g carbohydrates, 11 g fiber, 2 g total sugar, 12 g fat, 1.5 g saturated fat, 313 mg sodium, 334 mg potassium (10% DV), 66 mg calcium (7% DV), 55 mg magnesium (14% DV), 0 mcg B12 (0% DV), 0.16 mg B6 (8% DV), 2.5 mg iron (14% DV)

# Lentil and Pumpkin Soup

You might not assume that some of the spices used in this dish would pair well with savory flavors, but they SO do. By using sweeter spices like cinnamon and nutmeg, the natural sweetness of the pumpkin is enhanced, so there's less of a need for heartburn triggers like garlic and onion, and even less for gobs of salt. The sodium stats on a hefty portion of this soup are around half that of a much smaller portion of many store-bought or restaurant soups.

makes 4 servings (about 1½ cups per serving) / prep time: 10 minutes / total time: 50 minutes

2 tablespoons coconut oil

1 large carrot, chopped

1 large celery stalk, chopped

1 small shallot, chopped

2 cups orange or red lentils

½ teaspoon coarse sea salt

½ teaspoon ground coriander

Pinch of ground nutmeg

Pinch of ground cloves

Pinch of ground cinnamon

4 cups vegetable or chicken broth

2 cups water

1 (15 ounce) can 100% pure pumpkin puree

Heat the oil in a large pot or Dutch oven over medium heat. Add the carrot, celery, and shallot and cook until tender, but not browned, about 10 minutes. Add the lentils, salt, coriander, nutmeg, cloves, and cinnamon and cook, stirring, for an additional minute.

Pour in the broth, water, and pumpkin and bring to a boil. Reduce to a simmer, cover, and cook, stirring every 5 to 10 minutes, until the lentils are soft and starting to fall apart, about 30 minutes.

Per serving: 489 calories, 31 g protein, 74 g carbohydrates, 15 g fiber, 6 g total sugar, 11 g fat, 2.0 g saturated fat, 252 mg sodium, 1149 mg potassium (33% DV), 99 mg calcium (10% DV), 107 mg magnesium (27% DV), 0.24 mcg B12 (4% DV), 0.551 mg B6 (28% DV), 9.7 mg iron (54% DV)

# Zucchini, Mushroom, and Chicken Farfalle

You know the recipes that you can always count on if you need to impress or suddenly find yourself with hungry, unexpected guests? This is one of those recipes, because it's a true crowd-pleaser. It's got pasta, but there are more veggies and chicken than pasta, so it's a dish that will leave you feeling satisfied and energized. The thyme pairs perfectly with the mushrooms and chicken and gives this dish a cozy, home-cooked Sunday night dinner around the family table vibe.

makes 4 servings / prep time: 10 minutes / total time: 20 minutes

**2 cups dry whole grain farfalle (bow-tie) pasta**

**4 tablespoons olive oil, divided**

**2 cups sliced mushrooms**

**2 cups sliced zucchini**

**1 tablespoon chopped shallot**

**2 teaspoons dried thyme**

**½ teaspoon coarse sea salt**

**1 pound skinless, boneless chicken thighs, coarsely chopped**

Prepare the pasta according to the package directions.

Heat 2 tablespoons of the oil in a large skillet over medium-high heat. Add the mushrooms, zucchini, and shallot and sauté until tender and golden brown, about 10 minutes. Add 1 tablespoon of the oil, the thyme, salt, and chicken and cook until the chicken is cooked through and lightly browned, about 6 minutes.

Add the remaining 1 tablespoon oil to the skillet along with the cooked pasta and toss gently. Remove from the heat and serve.

Per serving: 452 calories, 34 g protein, 43 g carbohydrates, 6 g fiber, 2 g total sugar, 18 g fat, 2.5 g saturated fat, 283 mg sodium, 805 mg potassium (23% DV), 51 mg calcium (5% DV), 120 mg magnesium (3% DV), 0.241 mcg B12 (4% DV), 1.107 mg B6 (55% DV), 3.7 mg iron (20% DV)

> Shallots deliver a flavor somewhere between a mild onion and garlic and can be better tolerated than onions and garlic by some people with heartburn. If you are missing onion terribly, try adding cooked shallot to a meal to see if it works for you.

# Zucchini Stuffed with Thanksgiving

What's a girl with heartburn gotta do to get a little flavor into her meals? Stuff them with Thanksgiving. This meal manages to pack in major flavor, yet none of the typical heartburn triggers (ahem, onions . . .) are anywhere to be found. Plus, you get a major veggie boost (2 servings) with each portion.

makes 4 servings (2 zucchini halves per serving) / prep time: 30 minutes / total time: 1 hour

**4 large zucchini**

**1 tablespoon olive oil**

**12 ounces ground turkey breast**

**1 teaspoon coarse sea salt, divided**

**1½ cups cooked wild rice**

**½ cup dried cranberries**

**½ cup chopped toasted pecans**

**½ teaspoon dried oregano**

**½ teaspoon dried sage**

**½ teaspoon dried thyme**

Preheat the oven to 400°F. Cut each zucchini in half lengthwise and gently scrape out the seeds. Reserve the seeds. Place the zucchini halves on a baking sheet and bake until they begin to get tender, about 30 minutes.

Cook the zucchini seeds in the oil in a skillet over medium-high heat until soft, about 10 minutes. Add the turkey and ½ teaspoon of the salt and cook, breaking up the meat with a wooden spoon, until crumbled and browned and the zucchini seeds are golden, another 10 minutes. Set aside to cool slightly.

In a medium bowl, combine the cooled zucchini seeds and turkey mixture with the wild rice, cranberries, pecans, remaining ½ teaspoon salt, oregano, sage, and thyme. Place the pre-baked zucchini into a baking dish, scooped out indentations facing up, with about ¼ cup of water on the bottom of the dish. Position the zucchini next to one another, with their edges touching. Fill the indentations with the turkey mixture, heaping it high and spreading it across the rows of zucchini. Bake until the zucchini is fork-tender and the turkey filling is piping hot, about 25 minutes more.

Per serving: 410 calories, 23 g protein, 35 g carbohydrates, 6 g fiber, 18 g total sugar, 22 g fat, 3.5 g saturated fat, 650 mg sodium, 1126 mg potassium (32% DV), 92 mg calcium (9% DV), 117 mg magnesium (29% DV), 1.021 mcg B12 (17% DV), 0.93 mg B6 (47% DV), 3 mg iron (17% DV)

Healthy, Happy Pregnancy Cookbook

# Ginger-Soy Chia Chickpea Veggie Burgers

Veggie burgers so often come along with the usual suspects of acid reflux: onion, garlic, tomato, black pepper. Not these guys! These delicious burgers are loaded with flavor, packed with nutrition, take 15 minutes to make, and won't trigger that terrible burn. Now, if only they'd clean your kitchen for you, too.

makes 4 servings / prep time: 10 minutes / total time: 25 minutes

**2 (15-ounce) cans chickpeas, rinsed and drained, divided**

**⅓ cup water**

**¼ cup chia seeds**

**2 tablespoons reduced-sodium soy sauce**

**1 tablespoon sweet white miso paste**

**2 teaspoons minced fresh ginger**

**2 tablespoons olive oil, plus 2 teaspoons**

**½ cup grated carrots**

**½ cup grated zucchini**

**¼ teaspoon sea salt**

**½ teaspoon ground cumin**

**½ cup whole grain bread crumbs (see Note)**

In a small blender or food processor, blend 1 can of the chickpeas, the water, chia seeds, soy sauce, miso paste, and ginger until the beans are smooth (the chia seeds will remain whole), about 1½ minutes.

In a skillet, heat the 2 teaspoons oil over medium-high heat. Add the carrots and zucchini, sprinkle with the salt and cumin, and sauté until tender and golden, about 5 minutes. Stir the carrots, zucchini, and the remaining can of chickpeas into the pureed mixture. Stir until all the ingredients are evenly distributed. Stir in the bread crumbs until the mixture forms a ball.

Form the mixture into 4 large patties (or 6 medium patties) and sauté in a large skillet in the 2 tablespoons oil over medium heat until browned and crispy on both sides, 8 to 10 minutes total.

*Note:* You can also blend ¾ cup gluten-free old-fashioned rolled oats into a powder to use as a whole grain, gluten-free alternative.

Per serving: 388 calories, 15 g protein, 46 g carbohydrates, 15 g fiber, 7 g total sugar, 17 g fat, 2.0 g saturated fat, 520 mg sodium, 471 mg potassium (13% DV), 170 mg calcium (17% DV), 106 mg magnesium (27% DV), 0 mcg B12 (0% DV), 0.306 mg B6 (15% DV), 5 mg iron (28% DV)

# Soy-Sesame Scallop Stir-Fry

Stir-fries are typically loaded with garlic. And for good reason—it's delicious. This stir-fry is garlic-free and equally delicious . . . we promise! It's also a totally balanced meal all in one dish, with lean protein (thanks, scallops), healthy fats (take a bow, sesame and olive oils), veggies (you know who you are), and whole grains (will the brown jasmine rice please stand up?).

makes 4 servings / prep time: 10 minutes / total time: 30 minutes

**2 tablespoons olive oil, divided**

**4 cups cauliflower florets and stems cut into bite-size pieces**

**4 cups chopped bok choy**

**1 tablespoon toasted sesame oil**

**2½ teaspoons minced fresh ginger**

**2 tablespoons reduced-sodium soy sauce**

**1 pound sea scallops**

**4 cups cooked brown jasmine rice**

Heat 1 tablespoon of the olive oil in a very large skillet over medium heat. Add the cauliflower and sauté until golden and tender, about 15 minutes. Add the bok choy, sesame oil, ginger, and soy sauce and sauté until the bok choy leaves wilt but the stems are still firm, about 3 minutes. Remove the veggies from the pan and set aside on a plate.

Increase the heat to medium-high and add the remaining 1 tablespoon olive oil to the skillet. Add the scallops, spacing them evenly, and cook until opaque and firm and browned on each side, turning once, 5 to 6 minutes. Add the veggies back to the skillet and toss. Serve the stir-fry over the rice.

Per serving: 396 calories, 22 g protein, 57 g carbohydrates, 7 g fiber, 3 g total sugar, 9 g fat, 1.5 g saturated fat, 516 mg sodium, 892 mg potassium (25% DV), 127 mg calcium (13% DV), 143 mg magnesium (36% DV), 1.6 mcg B12 (27% DV), 0.752 mg B6 (38% DV), 2.7 mg iron (15% DV)

# Fiesta Corny Muffins

Cornbread goes with everything: salad, soup, and chili. It can even be the bread for a sandwich. Think of this corn muffin recipe as portion-controlled cornbread. Because it's packed with fun stuff like whole kernels of corn, spices, and bell peppers, it has more flavor and a more exciting texture than the classic recipe (no hate on the classic, though). It's also whole grain, which means that while you're enjoying all of that flavor, sans heartburn triggers, your body is benefitting from the extra fiber and nutrients that whole grains bring along.

makes 12 muffins / prep time: 10 minutes / total time: 35 minutes

**Olive oil spray**

**1 cup yellow cornmeal**

**¾ cup whole wheat flour**

**2 tablespoons sugar**

**1½ teaspoons baking powder**

**¾ teaspoon ground cumin**

**¾ teaspoon smoked paprika**

**½ teaspoon baking soda**

**¼ teaspoon coarse sea salt**

**1 cup corn kernels (fresh or frozen and thawed)**

**½ cup diced green bell peppers**

**1 cup low-fat milk or unsweetened dairy-free alternative**

**¼ cup coconut oil**

**1 tablespoon apple cider vinegar**

**2 large eggs**

Preheat the oven to 375°F. Coat a 12-cup muffin tin with olive oil spray.

In a large bowl, combine the cornmeal, flour, sugar, baking powder, cumin, paprika, baking soda, and salt. Stir in the corn and bell peppers. Set aside.

In a separate bowl, whisk the milk, oil, vinegar, and eggs. Pour the liquid mixture into the dry mixture and stir until all the dry ingredients are moistened. Do not overstir.

Fill each cup of the muffin tin evenly with batter. Bake until the tops are golden and the muffins are baked through, about 25 minutes.

Per serving: 148 calories, 4 g protein, 20 g carbohydrates, 3 g fiber, 3 g total sugar, 7 g fat, 4.5 g saturated fat, 306 mg sodium, 169 mg potassium (5% DV), 135 mg calcium (14% DV), 33 mg magnesium (8% DV), 0.197 mcg B12 (3% DV), 0.151 mg B6 (8% DV), 1.1 mg iron (6% DV)

# Fro-Ba (Frozen Banana "Ice Cream") with Peanut Butter Sauce

If you like the texture of soft-serve or fro-yo (probably safe to assume this is 99.9 percent of readers), then you will be happy to learn that you can make that deliciousness at home using a handful of ingredients that you probably already have. But unlike traditional ice cream, soft-serve, and fro-yo, this doesn't have any added sugar, is packed with vitamins, and even has protein and fiber for good measure. All we really needed to say was "peanut butter and banana," though, right? Elvis will be smiling down from heaven when you make this recipe.

makes 4 servings / prep time: 7 minutes + overnight / total time: 7 minutes

- **3 large very ripe bananas, cut into ¼-inch slices and frozen at least 4 hours (or overnight)**
- **2 tablespoons unsalted natural peanut butter**
- **3 tablespoons low-fat milk or unsweetened dairy-free alternative**
- **2 tablespoons chopped roasted peanuts**

Add the frozen bananas to a blender or food processor and pulse until they begin to crumble. If you're using a blender, you may need to use a spatula to push the bananas down in between pulses. Continue to pulse until the bananas start to look gooey, then turn the blender on and run until the mixture resembles soft-serve ice cream, about 3 minutes total.

Spoon the bananas into a freezer container and transfer to the freezer while you make the peanut sauce, or for at least 15 minutes.

Place the peanut butter and milk in a microwave-safe container and microwave on high for 20 seconds. Stir the mixture and microwave in 10-second increments, stirring in between, until the mixture is completely smooth, 30 to 40 seconds total.

Scoop the banana ice cream into 4 bowls, and top each with one-quarter of the peanut butter sauce and ½ tablespoon of the roasted peanuts.

Per serving: 164 calories, 4 g protein, 26 g carbohydrates, 3 g fiber, 14 g total sugar, 6 g fat, 1.0 g saturated fat, 4 mg sodium, 451 mg potassium (13% DV), 17 mg calcium (2% DV), 48 mg magnesium (12% DV), 0.017 mcg B12 (0% DV), 0.43 mg B6 (22% DV), 0.5 mg iron (3% DV)

## additional things you can do to reduce heartburn

- Eat smaller meals more frequently to avoid getting too full.
- Walk around or stand after each meal (maybe an evening walk after dinner?).
- Drink liquids between meals, not during them.
- Stay regular (see chapter 4).
- Wait at least an hour after eating dinner to go to bed.
- Consider propping your shoulders and head up with pillows when sleeping.

# CHAPTER FOUR

# Get a Move On: Recipes to Relieve/Prevent Constipation

Blame it on the hormones, because they're back at it. Hormones that help muscles to relax during pregnancy, which is necessary for delivery, also affect muscles of the intestinal system. Meaning, stuff is gonna take a little longer to move on through. As your abdomen becomes more crowded with baby this can put pressure on your gastrointestinal tract and slow things down even further. Also, the iron in your prenatal multivitamin and/or an additional iron supplement (if your doc recommended one) can be constipating. If it is, ask your doc to try a less constipating form of iron.

For eating to beat constipation, fiber (both soluble and insoluble) and magnesium are the key players in these recipes. Soluble fiber is the kind that dissolves into water and helps waste hold onto more water as it moves through your system, meaning smoother transit. Insoluble fiber doesn't dissolve in water and acts to add bulk to waste and speed up the travel time through your system. Both are important and both require plenty of water to work their magic. So, hear this PSA on hydration. Drink enough water all day long so that your pee is clear or very pale yellow, like lemonade. If your pee looks like apple juice . . . girl, you need to drink up.

And finally, these recipes contain foods with magnesium, a nutrient that helps attract water to the waste moving on through and helps it, well, move on through.

# Vanilla, Hazelnut, and Berry Baked Oatmeal

Get ready to impress family, guests, or fellow potluck brunchers with this dish. Most importantly, prepare to majorly impress yourself. Because this dish is based on whole grains (oats!) and gets flavor power from one of the most fiber-rich fruits (berries!) it packs a serious fiber punch into each serving. It also contains magnesium-rich hazelnuts, adding another level of smooth move power.

makes 6 servings / prep time: 5 minutes / total time: 1 hour 5 minutes

1 tablespoon coconut oil

2 cups old-fashioned rolled oats

1½ cups chopped toasted hazelnuts, divided

1½ teaspoons baking powder

¾ teaspoon ground cinnamon

2 cups low-fat milk or unsweetened dairy-free alternative

2 large eggs

2 tablespoons honey

2 tablespoons pure vanilla extract

4 cups fresh or frozen and thawed mixed berries (raspberries, strawberries, blueberries), divided

Preheat the oven to 375°F. Grease an 8 x 8-inch baking dish with the oil.

In a large bowl, stir together the oats, ½ cup of the hazelnuts, the baking powder, and cinnamon.

In a medium bowl, whisk the milk, eggs, honey, and vanilla.

Sprinkle 2 cups of the berries on the bottom of the dish followed by ½ cup of the hazelnuts. Sprinkle the oat mixture on next, making sure that it is evenly spread across the dish. Pour the milk mixture on top of the oats, pouring slowly and evenly to ensure that the milk soaks in and is distributed evenly. Top with the remaining 2 cups berries and remaining ½ cup hazelnuts.

Bake until firm with a golden top, about 55 minutes. Remove from the oven and let cool for 5 minutes before serving. You can eat it as is or top with yogurt, maple syrup, and/or a drizzle of milk. It's also really tasty served cold.

Per serving: 427 calories, 14 g protein, 42 g carbohydrates, 11 g fiber, 14 g total sugar, 15 g fat, 4.5 g saturated fat, 184 mg sodium, 578 mg potassium (17% DV), 245 mg calcium (25% DV), 115 mg magnesium (29% DV), 0.573 mcg B12 (10% DV), 0.289 mg B6 (14% DV), 3.6 mg iron (20% DV)

Healthy, Happy Pregnancy Cookbook

# Pear and Almond Butter–Stuffed French Toast

Stuffed French toast sounds super fancy and difficult, until you think of it as simply "French toast-ifying" a sandwich. Just don't tell the people you're serving how simple it really is. An added bonus to making restaurant-worthy brunch dishes at home—other than getting to stay in your PJs—is that you can use more nutritious ingredients, like whole grain bread, more spices and fruit, and a whole lot less sugar. This dish packs in the fiber and flavor without leaving you in a sugar-induced stupor.

makes 4 servings / prep time: 5 minutes / total time: 45 minutes

**6 teaspoons creamy unsalted natural almond butter, divided**

**6 slices whole grain bread**

**2 medium pears, thinly sliced**

**2 large eggs**

**½ cup 1% milk or soy milk**

**½ large very ripe banana, mashed smooth**

**1 teaspoon ground ginger**

**1 tablespoon finely grated lemon zest**

**½ teaspoon pure vanilla extract**

**1 tablespoon unsalted butter**

**½ cup low-fat plain Greek yogurt**

**2 tablespoons pure maple syrup**

Spread 1 teaspoon of the almond butter onto each slice of bread. Top the almond butter on three of the slices with one-third of the sliced pears. Top each of the pear-topped slices with the remaining 3 almond butter–covered slices, almond butter side facing the pear mixture. Press down very firmly to seal the two halves together.

Whisk the eggs, milk, banana, ginger, lemon zest, and vanilla in a large glass measuring cup. Pour into a deep pie plate. Dip each pear-almond butter sandwich into the egg mixture, allowing the egg to soak in on each side.

Heat the butter in a large skillet over medium heat. Cook the egg-soaked sandwiches until golden brown and the bread is firm, 2 to 2½ minutes per side. Cut each into quarters. Stir the maple syrup into the yogurt in a small bowl. Top each serving (3 quarters) of the French toast with 2 tablespoons of the yogurt mixture and additional maple syrup to taste.

Per serving: 378 calories, 9 g protein, 57 g carbohydrates, 10 g fiber, 24 g total sugar, 12 g fat, 4 g saturated fat, 222 mg sodium, 313 mg potassium (9% DV), 193 mg calcium (19% DV), 40 mg magnesium (1% DV), 0.372 mcg B12 (6% DV), 0.14 mg B6 (7% DV), 2.6 mg iron (15% DV)

# Asparagus and White Bean Strata

Imagine a slice of grainy toast topped with scrambled eggs, roasted veggies, and a sprinkle of cheese. A strata is a casserole version of that toast you just imagined, and it doesn't disappoint. The fact that it can be made the night before makes it a convenient way to have a hot, homemade, fancy schmancy breakfast in the morning. And this strata is especially impressive because it not only tastes amazing, it also supplies major soluble and insoluble fiber benefits as well as magnesium.

makes 6 servings / prep time: 30 minutes / total time: 1 hour 55 minutes + overnight

1 large onion, sliced

4 teaspoons olive oil, divided

1 pound asparagus, ends trimmed, coarsely chopped

½ teaspoon coarse sea salt

¼ teaspoon freshly ground black pepper

1 (15-ounce) can white beans, rinsed and drained, divided

1 cup low-fat milk or dairy-free alternative

6 large eggs

2 tablespoons ground flaxseeds

¼ teaspoon ground nutmeg

6 slices whole grain bread, cut in half diagonally

1 cup shredded part-skim mozzarella cheese or dairy-free alternative, divided

In a large skillet over medium heat, cook the onion in 3 teaspoons of the oil until it begins to soften, about 10 minutes. Add the asparagus, salt, and pepper and cook until the asparagus softens and the onion is golden, about 8 minutes more.

Puree half of the beans in a blender or food processor with the milk. In a medium bowl, whisk the eggs, flaxseeds, nutmeg, and pureed beans. Set aside.

Oil an 8 x 8-inch baking dish with the remaining 1 teaspoon oil. Arrange the bread slices in the baking dish so that they completely cover the bottom, overlapping the slices so they all fit.

Sprinkle the remaining whole beans over the bread layer and sprinkle on ½ cup of the cheese. Spread the asparagus-onion mixture evenly over the top. Slowly pour the egg and pureed bean mixture over the top, giving it time to soak into each layer. Sprinkle the top with the remaining ½ cup cheese. Cover the strata with plastic wrap and refrigerate for 4 hours or overnight.

Preheat the oven to 350°F. Remove the strata from the fridge and allow to sit at room temperature while the oven preheats. Place the baking dish of strata onto a baking sheet (to catch any potential spillover during baking) and bake until firm and golden, about 1 hour 15 minutes. Let cool for 15 minutes before serving to allow the strata to firm up.

Per serving: 406 calories, 21 g protein, 46 g carbohydrates, 10 g fiber, 9 g total sugar, 15 g fat, 5 g saturated fat, 402 mg sodium, 733 mg potassium (21% DV), 363 mg calcium (36% DV), 79 mg magnesium (20% DV), 1.348 mcg B12 (22% DV), 0.277 mg B6 (14% DV), 6.1 mg iron (34% DV)

## probiotics during pregnancy?

Probiotics from supplements and fermented foods are hotter than a shirtless Channing Tatum right now (queue collective sigh). They deserve the attention—these good-for-you bacteria that reside in your gut are being linked to a growing list of health benefits for you and baby, including a potential reduction in risk for preterm labor and allergies. Eating naturally fiber-rich foods, including vegetarian meals on a regular basis, limiting highly processed foods, managing stress, and staying active can all help nourish the friendly bacteria you already have residing in your gut and encourage more to set up shop. Fermented foods, like sauerkraut, kombucha, yogurt, kefir, and kimchi can also help to populate your gut with the friendly critters. Unlike supplements, fermented foods also bring along additional nutrients. Sauerkraut and kimchi deliver antioxidant- and fiber-packed veggie servings, yogurt provides protein and calcium, and kombucha hydrates. Probiotic supplements are also an option, though supplement quality and effectiveness can vary a lot depending on the manufacturer, and it's important to talk to your doctor or midwife about which specific strains of bacteria are right for you. When making a decision about probiotic-rich foods or supplements, make sure you trust the company to provide a safe product. For supplements, we like VSL #3, Culturelle, and Align, but there are plenty of good options out there. Ask your doctor/midwife which brands they prefer. The bottom line is that there are enough potential benefits from probiotics during pregnancy to merit including them in your routine. We recommend food sources over supplements whenever possible, but no matter how you choose to get your probiotics, do your research to find products/brands that are trustworthy.

# Chocolate Breakfast Milk Shake

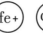

Not only does it taste like you're having a milk shake for breakfast, but this smoothie also hydrates, contains magnesium, and packs in well over half of your daily fiber needs. Win-win! It also contains bananas, which have probiotic substances, stuff that your natural, good gut bacteria love to feast on and can help keep the good bacteria healthy and happy.

makes 2 meal-size servings, or 4 snack-size servings / prep time: 5 minutes / total time: 5 minutes

**2½ cups steamed cauliflower florets and stems, cooled (see Note)**

**3 large ripe bananas**

**2 cups unsweetened almond milk**

**1½ cups cubed silken or soft tofu (about 5 ounces)**

**3 to 4 tablespoons unsweetened cocoa powder (depending on how chocolaty you want it . . . we use 4)**

**1 tablespoon tahini**

**1 cup ice cubes**

**2 tablespoons cacao nibs**

Place the cauliflower, bananas, milk, tofu, cocoa powder, and tahini in a blender and blend on high until smooth, about 1½ minutes. Add the ice and blend until it's incorporated, about 1 minute more. Top each serving with 1 tablespoon of the cacao nibs.

*Note:* The cauliflower can be steamed in advance and refrigerated until needed.

Per serving: 367 calories, 15 g protein, 61 g carbohydrates, 17 g fiber, 25 g total sugar, 18 g fat, 4 g saturated fat, 254 mg sodium, 1337 mg potassium (38% DV), 591 mg calcium (59% DV), 114 mg magnesium (29% DV), 0 mcg B12 (0% DV), 0.948 mg B6 (47% DV), 4.2 mg iron (24% DV)

Healthy, Happy Pregnancy Cookbook

# Fajita-Style Breakfast Burrito

These burritos are packed with flavor and a combination of protein, healthy fat, and fiber that keeps you satisfied well into the morning. You can even wrap them in plastic wrap and aluminum foil and freeze them for mornings when you need to unwrap, nuke, and go.

makes 4 servings / prep time: 5 minutes / total time: 15 minutes

2 tablespoons olive oil, divided

1 medium onion, chopped

2 cups sliced cremini or white mushrooms

1 green bell pepper, chopped

1 red bell pepper, chopped

¼ teaspoon coarse sea salt

⅛ teaspoon ground cumin

⅛ teaspoon ground coriander

⅛ teaspoon garlic powder

6 large eggs

½ cup salsa

4 (10-inch) whole grain tortillas

In a large skillet, heat 1 tablespoon of the oil over medium heat and sauté the onion until it just begins to turn translucent, about 4 minutes. Add the mushrooms, bell peppers, salt, cumin, coriander, and garlic powder and continue to cook until the onion and mushrooms are golden, the peppers are soft, and there's no excess liquid from the veggies left in the pan, about 8 minutes more. Set the mixture aside.

Whisk together the eggs and salsa. Cook in the remaining 1 tablespoon oil in a medium skillet over medium heat until firm, stirring occasionally, about 2 minutes.

Place one-quarter of the egg mixture onto each of the 4 tortillas. Top each with one-quarter of the veggie mixture. Fold both ends of each tortilla in and roll up.

Per serving: 383 calories, 17 g protein, 40 g carbohydrates, 7 g fiber, 6 g total sugar, 19 g fat, 4 g saturated fat, 662 mg sodium, 627 mg potassium (18% DV), 75 mg calcium (8% DV), 69 mg magnesium (17% DV), 0.981 mcg B12 (16% DV), 0.534 mg B6 (27% DV), 3.7 mg iron (21% DV)

# Barley Crab Cakes

These crab cakes are probably not like any you've seen or tasted before. Unique crab cake ingredients like veggies and barley lend a different but delicious flavor and texture, plus added fiber. Traditional crab cakes need to be paired with high-fiber carbs and veggies in order to be a balanced meal. With these cakes, you get all of those things built into one. Just serve with some additional veggies and your meal is done.

makes 4 servings (2 cakes each) / prep time: 10 minutes / total time: 30 minutes

**6 teaspoons olive oil, divided**

**½ cup shredded carrots**

**½ cup shredded zucchini**

**½ cup shredded onion**

**½ teaspoon sweet paprika**

**½ teaspoon ground turmeric**

**½ teaspoon coarse sea salt**

**¼ teaspoon freshly ground black pepper**

**2 large eggs**

**3 (6-ounce) cans lump crabmeat, drained and flaked**

**2 cups cooked barley**

**½ cup whole grain bread crumbs**

Heat 2 teaspoons of the oil in a large skillet over medium heat. Add the carrots, zucchini, onion, paprika, turmeric, salt, and pepper and sauté until soft and golden, about 5 minutes. Set aside.

In a large bowl, beat the eggs with a fork until blended. Stir in the crabmeat and vegetable mixture. Add the barley and stir until it is totally incorporated. Add the bread crumbs and stir until the mixture begins to stick together. Form the crabmeat mixture into 8 patties, squeezing each with firm pressure so it holds together.

Heat the remaining 4 teaspoons oil in the same skillet used for cooking the veggies over medium-high heat. Cook the crab cakes in the skillet until browned on each side, about 4 minutes per side.

Per serving: 361 calories, 27 g protein, 37 g carbohydrates, 6 g fiber, 5 g total sugar, 12 g fat, 2 g saturated fat, 597 mg sodium, 687 mg potassium (20% DV), 161 mg calcium (16% DV), 71 mg magnesium (18% DV), 0.754 mcg B12 (13% DV), 0.404 mg B6 (20% DV), 3.5 mg iron (19% DV)

# Chicken and Barley with Kale-Walnut Pesto

Pesto is delicious, but tends to be salty and heavy. This pesto is packed with kale, which has some veggie volume to it so you can eat a larger portion of food without feeling like you have a rock in your stomach. And instead of pasta, this dish uses barley, which adds a mega fiber boost.

makes 4 servings / prep time: 15 minutes / total time: 55 minutes

1 cup hulled barley

2½ cups water

4 bone-in, skin-on chicken thighs

Pesto

3 cups chopped kale leaves (tough ribs removed)

4 large fresh basil leaves

¼ cup walnuts

2 tablespoons olive oil

1½ garlic cloves

3 tablespoons water

½ teaspoon coarse sea salt or kosher salt

Pinch of freshly ground black pepper

1 teaspoon freshly squeezed lemon juice

Preheat the oven to 425°F. Line a baking dish with aluminum foil.

Bring the barley and the 2½ cups water to a boil in a large saucepan. Reduce to a simmer and cook, covered, until all the liquid is absorbed, about 40 minutes.

Place the chicken thighs, skin side up, in the baking dish. Reduce the temperature to 375°F and bake the chicken thighs until their internal temperature registers 165°F, about 30 minutes. Remove from the oven and let rest for 5 minutes.

Cook the kale in a large pot of boiling water until it just wilts, about 2 minutes. Drain and plunge into a large bowl of ice water. Once cooled, drain well.

Put the kale and the remaining ingredients, basil through lemon juice, in a small blender or food processor and blend on high until smooth, adding more water if needed.

Remove the skin from each thigh. Place ¾ cup of the cooked barley on each plate and top with 1 tablespoon of the pesto. Then place a chicken thigh onto the pesto and top with another tablespoon of pesto. Freeze or refrigerate the remaining ½ cup pesto.

Per serving: 499 calories, 30 g protein, 35 g carbohydrates, 8 g fiber, 0 g total sugar, 27 g fat, 7 g saturated fat, 139 mg sodium, 528 mg potassium (15% DV), 32 mg calcium (3% DV), 92 mg magnesium (23% DV), 0.954 mcg B12 (16% DV), 0.67 mg B6 (34% DV), 2.7 mg iron (15% DV)

# Green Lentil and Kabocha Squash Stew

Lentils should be the star of the next superhero movie, because they're pretty amazing. They could rid Gotham of constipation in no time. Not only are they packed with iron and protein, they are LOADED with fiber and also drag some magnesium along wherever they go. This stew is easy to make and has a great flavor payoff that completely belies its ease.

makes 4 servings / prep time: 10 minutes / total time: 1 hour 10 minutes

**1 medium onion, diced**

**3 tablespoons sunflower seed oil, divided**

**2 garlic cloves, minced**

**2 large tomatoes, diced**

**1 teaspoon minced fresh ginger**

**1 tablespoon tomato paste**

**1 teaspoon coarse sea salt**

**1 teaspoon ground turmeric**

**2 teaspoons curry powder (optional)**

**1 cup green lentils**

**4½ cups water, plus more as needed**

**1 small kabocha squash (about 2 pounds), cut into ½-inch dice, but not peeled (see Note)**

In a Dutch oven or very large skillet over medium heat, sauté the onion in 1 tablespoon of the oil until soft and golden, about 8 minutes. Add the remaining 2 tablespoons oil and the garlic and sauté until the garlic turns golden, about 1 minute more. Add the tomatoes, ginger, tomato paste, salt, and turmeric and sauté an additional minute. If you're turning this dish into a curry, add the curry powder now.

Add the lentils to the skillet and stir to coat the lentils with the oil and aromatics. Pour in the water and bring the mixture to a boil. Reduce to a simmer and cook the mixture until the lentils are just barely tender, 25 to 30 minutes. Add the squash and continue to simmer until the squash is tender, another 25 to 30 minutes, adding additional water in ½-cup increments if needed.

*Note:* If you're hesitant to leave the skin on the squash, take our word for it—you'll love it! Not only does the skin add extra fiber and nutrients, but it tastes fantastic and contributes a really great texture to the dish.

Per serving: 375 calories, 16 g protein, 57 g carbohydrates, 20 g fiber, 10 g total sugar, 11 g fat, 1.5 g saturated fat, 303 mg sodium, 1587 mg potassium (45% DV), 116 mg calcium (12% DV), 109 mg magnesium (27% DV), 0 mcg B12 (0% DV), 0.768 mg B6 (38% DV), 6 mg iron (33% DV)

Healthy, Happy Pregnancy Cookbook

# Loaded Fries (#PutAnEggOnIt)

For those nights when all you want for dinner (or lunch) is a plate of fries, this recipe will make you very, very happy. The addition of sautéed spinach and fried eggs takes French fries to the meal-worthy level. And the potatoes and spinach both deliver magnesium to the nutrient profile of this nosh.

makes 2 servings / prep time: 15 minutes / total time: 40 minutes

1 large russet potato, scrubbed but not peeled

2 tablespoons olive oil, divided

½ teaspoon coarse sea salt, divided

¼ teaspoon chili powder

¼ teaspoon garlic powder

⅛ teaspoon freshly ground black pepper

4 cups baby spinach

4 large eggs

Preheat the oven to 450°F.

Slice the potato lengthwise into ¼-inch slices. Then slice each of those lengthwise into ¼-inch square fry-shaped rods. Toss with 1 tablespoon of the oil, ¼ teaspoon of the salt, the chili powder, garlic powder, and pepper.

Arrange the potato sticks on a baking sheet so they aren't touching and bake until golden and crispy, about 30 minutes, turning once.

In a medium skillet over medium heat, sauté the spinach in ½ tablespoon of the oil until wilted, about 4 minutes. Sprinkle with the remaining ¼ teaspoon salt and set aside.

In the same skillet, add the remaining ½ tablespoon oil and cook eggs to your preferred doneness. Divide the fries between 2 plates and top each plate with half the spinach and 2 eggs.

Per serving: 422 calories, 18 g protein, 36 g carbohydrates, 4 g fiber, 2 g total sugar, 24 g fat, 5 g saturated fat, 477 mg sodium, 1238 mg potassium (35% DV), 137 mg calcium (14% DV), 102 mg magnesium (26% DV), 1.29 mcg B12 (22% DV), 0.897 mg B6 (45% DV), 5.1 mg iron (28% DV)

# Citrus-Thyme Cod over Millet

A flavorful and simple fish dish is nice to have in the cooking repertoire, especially when it uses the broiler and is ready in 20 minutes. This dish combines the fresh flavors of citrus with garlic and thyme to deliver a lot of flavor but with a lightness. And if you haven't tried millet yet, prepare to be amazed at how light and fluffy this whole grain is. Don't be fooled, though, it still packs fiber punch.

makes 4 servings / prep time: 10 minutes / total time: 20 minutes

**1 cup millet**

**2 cups water**

**2 tablespoons olive oil, plus 2 teaspoons**

**1 teaspoon finely grated lemon zest**

**1 teaspoon finely grated orange zest**

**1 tablespoon freshly squeezed lemon juice**

**1 tablespoon freshly squeezed orange juice**

**2 garlic cloves, minced**

**¾ teaspoon dried thyme**

**½ teaspoon coarse sea salt, divided**

**1 pound cod fillets**

**Pinch of freshly ground black pepper**

In a medium saucepan, bring the millet and water to a boil. Reduce to a simmer, cover, and continue cooking until the water is absorbed, 12 to 15 minutes. Set aside.

Preheat the broiler to high.

Whisk together the 2 tablespoons oil, the citrus zests, juices, garlic, thyme, and ¼ teaspoon of the salt.

Place the fish in a small baking dish in a single layer. Pour the oil mixture over the top of the fillets. Broil on high until the fish is firm and cooked through, about 6 minutes.

Toss the millet with the 2 teaspoons oil, ⅛ teaspoon of the salt, and the pinch of pepper. Sprinkle the fish with the remaining ⅛ teaspoon salt. Serve the fillets over the millet, and drizzle with the oil mixture remaining in the baking dish.

Per serving: 356 calories, 26 g protein, 38 g carbohydrates, 6 g fiber, 0 g total sugar, 11 g fat, 1.5 g saturated fat, 267 mg sodium, 491 mg potassium (14% DV), 39 mg calcium (39% DV), 90 mg magnesium (23% DV), 0 mcg B12 (0% DV), 0.215 mg B6 (11% DV), 2.1 mg iron (12% DV)

# Sun-Dried Tomato and Tuna Linguine

This is a very deceptive dish because it looks and tastes like you spent a loooooong time making it, but you so did not. A big bowl of pasta isn't typically the most soothing to a constipation situation, but this dish is different. The whole grain pasta adds fiber while together with the tuna and tomatoes it creates a magnesium trifecta. You will not be missing out on flavor with this dish, either, even though it has less sodium than a dish a quarter of its size from a restaurant.

makes 4 servings / prep time: 5 minutes / total time: 25 minutes

1 cup unsalted sun-dried tomatoes

8 ounces dry whole grain linguine

3 garlic cloves, sliced

2 tablespoons olive oil

2 (5-ounce) cans tuna packed in olive oil, very lightly drained

¼ teaspoon coarse sea salt

¼ cup chopped fresh chives

Soak the sun-dried tomatoes in warm water until they soften, about 10 minutes. Drain and slice into strips.

Meanwhile, cook the linguine according to the package directions. Drain.

In a large skillet, heat the oil over medium heat and sauté the garlic until golden, about 2 minutes. Add the sun-dried tomatoes, cooked pasta, tuna, and the salt. Reduce the heat to low and gently toss until all the ingredients are well distributed and warmed through, about 3 minutes.

Sprinkle each serving with 1 tablespoon of the chives.

Per serving: 409 calories, 27 g protein, 51 g carbohydrates, 8 g fiber, 5 g total sugar, 13 g fat, 2 g saturated fat, 240 mg sodium, 726 mg potassium (21% DV), 52 mg calcium (5% DV), 127 mg magnesium (32% DV), 1.247 mcg B12 (21% DV), 0.257 mg B6 (13% DV), 4.2 mg iron (24% DV)

# Buddha Bowl with Crispy Tofu

Buddha bowls come in all varieties of toppings and grains, but the one thing that ties them all together is that they're a deliciously satisfying meal in a bowl. This bowl uses farro, which is an ancient form of wheat in its least processed form. It's got a hearty texture and mega-fiber power. Aside from the flavorful soy-sesame-tahini sauce, the colorful broccoli, carrots, and purple cabbage make it is so darn pretty that it surely deserves a snapshot (not that you weren't going to take a picture of your food anyway!).

makes 4 servings / prep time: 10 minutes / total time: 55 minutes

1 (14-ounce) package firm tofu, drained weight

1 tablespoon olive oil

1 cup farro

4 cups water

3 cups broccoli florets and stems, cut into bite-size pieces

1½ cups packed carrot ribbons or grated carrots

1½ cups coarsely chopped red cabbage (bite-size pieces)

½ cup rice vinegar

3½ tablespoons reduced-sodium soy sauce

2 tablespoons toasted sesame oil

2 tablespoons tahini

1 tablespoon honey

2 teaspoons grated fresh ginger

Preheat the oven to 350°F.

Cut the tofu into 1-inch cubes and toss with the olive oil on a rimmed baking sheet. Spread out the tofu so that the cubes aren't touching. Bake until the tofu is golden and crispy on the outside, about 40 minutes, turning once.

In a medium saucepan, bring the farro and water to a boil. Reduce to a simmer, cover, and cook until the farro is tender, about 30 minutes. Drain excess water and set the farro aside.

Bring a large saucepan of water to a boil. Add the broccoli and cook just until the broccoli becomes a vivid green, about 2 minutes. Remove the broccoli and place it into a large bowl of ice water. Reserve the boiling water. Remove the cooled broccoli from the ice water and set aside.

Add the carrots to the boiling water and continue to boil until their color becomes more vivid, about 1 minute. Remove the carrots with a slotted spoon and plunge into the ice bath. Reserve the boiling water. Remove the carrots from ice bath and set aside. Repeat the process with the cabbage, cooking for 1 minute, and then submerging in the ice water.

*Healthy, Happy Pregnancy Cookbook*

Whisk together the vinegar, soy sauce, sesame oil, tahini, honey, and ginger.

Divide the farro among 4 bowls. Top the farro with one-quarter of the veggies and tofu, arranging them to each take up one-quarter of the top of the farro. Drizzle each bowl with one-quarter of the sauce.

Per serving: 451 calories, 21 g protein, 52 g carbohydrates, 9 g fiber, 13 g total sugar, 20 g fat, 3 g saturated fat, 569 mg sodium, 671 mg potassium (19% DV), 248 mg calcium (25% DV), 97 mg magnesium (24% DV), 0 mcg B12 (0% DV), 0.368 mg B6 (18% DV), 5.8 mg iron (32% DV)

# Sweet Potato Drop Biscuit–Topped Chicken Potpie

This dish combines two lovely foods, chicken stew and drop biscuits, into one incredible dish. It really should be called stewscuit, but let's just stick with potpie for now. Traditionally comforting foods like potpie are low in fiber. But, because this one has veggie-packed stew and a drop biscuit top made from whole grain flour and sweet potato, it makes a new (high fiber) name for potpie. This will quickly become a favorite. And, yes, if you ever need a quick drop biscuit recipe, you can totally make the biscuit portion of this recipe and bake sans stew.

makes 4 servings / prep time: 30 minutes / total time: 50 minutes

1 tablespoon olive oil

1 carrot, chopped

½ large yellow onion, chopped

1 celery stalk, chopped

½ cup sliced cremini mushrooms

½ cup peas (fresh or frozen)

1 pound boneless, skinless chicken breast, diced

½ teaspoon garlic powder

½ teaspoon ground cumin

½ teaspoon dried basil

¼ teaspoon coarse sea salt, plus a pinch

¼ teaspoon freshly ground black pepper

¼ teaspoon ground coriander

2 tablespoon whole wheat flour

1 cup low-sodium chicken broth

**Biscuits**

¾ cup whole wheat flour

2 teaspoons baking powder

¼ teaspoon coarse sea salt

4 tablespoons (½ stick) unsalted butter

½ cup mashed sweet potatoes (about 1 medium)

¼ cup low-fat milk or unsweetened dairy-free alternative

Preheat the oven to 425°F.

In a large oven-safe pot, such as a Dutch oven, heat the oil over medium-high heat. Sauté the carrot, onion, celery, mushrooms, and peas until tender and lightly browned, about 8 minutes. Add the chicken, garlic powder, cumin, basil, ¼ teaspoon salt, pepper, and coriander. Cook, stirring gently, until the chicken is just cooked through, about 7 minutes. Stir in the flour and continue

*Healthy, Happy Pregnancy Cookbook*

to cook, stirring, until all the liquid is incorporated and you can't see the flour anymore, about 1 minute. Add the broth and continue cooking and stirring until the mixture thickens, 3 to 4 minutes. Set aside.

Whisk together the flour, baking powder, and salt. Using a fork (or your hands—which is our preferred tool), mash the butter into the mixture until it looks like bread crumbs. Stir the sweet potato and milk together until smooth. Gently stir the sweet potato mixture into the flour mixture until well combined; the dough will be sticky. Place one-quarter of the dough onto each quarter of the surface of the chicken mixture, making sure that the dough doesn't overlap with the neighboring quarter of dough.

Bake until the biscuits are fluffy and golden, about 24 minutes.

Per serving: 422 calories, 31 g protein, 34 g carbohydrates, 6 g fiber, 6 g total sugar, 19 g fat, 9 g saturated fat, 564 mg sodium, 894 mg potassium (26% DV), 204 mg calcium (20% DV), 90 mg magnesium (23% DV), 0.356 mcg B12 (6% DV), 1.133 mg B6 (57% DV), 2.4 mg iron (13% DV)

# Vanilla-Pumpkin Hummus

Dipping foods is fun. It just is. You can take the same ingredients and eat them in a bunch of other delightful ways, but once you get to dip sweet slices of pear into a creamy, vanilla-laden dip, you've found your snack time winner. This dip makes a great snack because it's made from chickpeas, which means that it delivers fiber and protein in each bite. It's also so delicious and fun to eat that you'll want to make a big batch and use it for snacks all week long (which is highly recommended).

makes 4 servings / prep time: 5 minutes / total time: 5 minutes

**1 cup rinsed and drained chickpeas**

**½ cup canned 100% pure pumpkin puree**

**1 teaspoon pure vanilla extract**

**1 tablespoon tahini**

**1 tablespoon sunflower seed oil**

**1 tablespoon pure maple syrup**

**Pinch of ground cinnamon**

**3 to 4 tablespoons skim milk or unsweetened dairy-free alternative**

**1 pear, divided**

**2 tablespoons chopped toasted pecans**

Puree the chickpeas, pumpkin, vanilla, tahini, oil, maple syrup, and cinnamon in a small blender or food processor, adding 1 tablespoon of milk at a time until you reach the desired consistency (3 to 4 tablespoons total).

Finely chop one-third of the pear and gently stir it into the hummus. Slice the remaining pear. Top the hummus with pecans and serve with the pear slices. This is also a great dip for celery and carrot sticks!

Per serving: 180 calories, 4 g protein, 22 g carbohydrates, 7 g fiber, 8 g total sugar, 9 g fat, 1 g saturated fat, 87 mg sodium, 195 mg potassium (6% DV), 50 mg calcium (5% DV), 28 mg magnesium (7% DV), 0 mcg B12 (0% DV), 0.042 mg B6 (2% DV), 1.4 mg iron (8% DV)

# Sweet and Salty Popcorn Trail Mix

Trail mix is delicious, fun to eat, and satisfying. The major downside to trail mix (womp, womp . . .) is that it's WAY too easy to down a giant portion, only to realize that you've eaten enough to count for your intended snack plus a large dinner. This trail mix is based on freshly popped popcorn, so you get a big ol' portion. Its flavor comes from cinnamon (which brings out the natural sweetness in the other ingredients without the need to add sweetener), pistachios, and dried cherries. All of these ingredients deliver flavor, texture, and antioxidants. They're multitaskers, just like you.

makes 4 servings / prep time: 5 minutes / total time: 5 minutes

**¼ cup popcorn kernels**

**1 tablespoon coconut oil**

**1 teaspoon ground cinnamon**

**⅓ cup roasted and salted shelled pistachios**

**⅓ cup dried cherries**

Combine the popcorn kernels and oil in a large saucepan with a tight-fitting lid. Toss gently to coat the kernels with the oil. Place the pan, with the lid on, over high heat and wait for popping sounds to start.

Once the popping begins to slow down to about a pop every 2 seconds, about 2½ minutes after putting it on the burner, remove the pan from heat and pour the popped kernels into a large bowl. Toss the popcorn with the cinnamon to coat, and then gently toss with pistachios and cherries.

Per serving: 148 calories, 3 g protein, 17 g carbohydrates, 3 g fiber, 7 g total sugar, 8 g fat, 3.5 g saturated fat, 45 mg sodium, 136 mg potassium (4% DV), 24 mg magnesium (6% DV), 19 mg calcium (2% DV), 0 mcg B12 (0% DV), 0.132 mg B6 (7% DV), 0.8 mg iron (4% DV)

# CHAPTER FIVE

# My Calves Are in a Knot: Recipes to Help Ease and Prevent Leg Cramps

Leg cramps most commonly appear during the second and third trimesters. If you've had one, you know it's no picnic.

Here's a common scenario: You've finally found a comfy position to get to sleep, and just as you drift off, BAM, your calf muscle is contracting like a boa constrictor. The cramp delivers the kind of jolt that requires a yelp, which wakes up your partner for the third time this week asking, "Is it time?"

The best thing to do to treat leg cramps is to help prevent them. There are important non-dietary things you can do, such as not sitting in one position for long periods of time, stretching your calves often, and remaining active. In terms of diet, staying hydrated and getting a few key nutrients that play a role in muscle contraction, including potassium, magnesium, and calcium, can help prevent cramping.

This chapter is loaded with foods rich in all of these nutrients and with a higher percentage of water, so you're getting more hydration without even drinking.

# Blueberry-Banana Oat Smoothie

The classic combination of berries and banana is always a palate pleaser and you'll never know you snuck in a serving of veggies at breakfast! Banana and spinach contribute potassium to help ease cramping, while blueberries pack in fiber and antioxidants for an additional health boost and milk provides a hefty dose of magnesium.

makes 1 serving / prep time: 5 minutes / total time: 5 minutes

1 cup 1% milk or unsweetened dairy-free alternative

1 cup baby spinach leaves

½ large very ripe banana, cut into chunks and frozen overnight

1 cup blueberries (fresh or frozen)

1 tablespoon unsalted natural almond butter

½ cup ice cubes (if using fresh berries)

Combine the milk and spinach in a blender and blend on high until smooth, 1 to 1½ minutes. Add the banana, blueberries, and almond butter and blend again until smooth, about 1½ minutes more. If using fresh berries, add the ice and blend again until smooth, about 30 seconds.

Per serving: 355 calories, 13 g protein, 54 g carbohydrates, 6.5 g fiber, 37 g total sugar, 13 g fat, 2.5 g saturated fat, 205 mg sodium, 1012 mg potassium (29% DV), 390 mg calcium (39% DV), 126 mg magnesium (32% DV), 1.1 mcg B12 (19% DV), 0.5 mg B6 (24% DV), 2 mg iron (11% DV)

# Orange-Carrot Cream Smoothie

Creamy and bursting with orange flavor, this smoothie reminds us of Creamsicles from childhood. In addition to helping with hydration, the yogurt in this smoothie packs in magnesium to help prevent cramping.

makes 1 serving / prep time: 5 minutes / total time: 5 minutes

½ cup shredded or chopped carrots

1 small orange, peeled and divided into segments

1 cup low-fat plain yogurt

¼ cup freshly squeezed orange juice

5 almonds

1 cup ice cubes

Combine the carrots, orange segments, yogurt, orange juice, almonds, and ice in a blender. Blend on high until smooth, 30 to 60 seconds.

*Note:* Smoothies are a great make-ahead breakfast. Whip up a batch or two the night before, and then refrigerate in a sealed single-serving container (mason jars are perfectly portable). In the morning, stir, and it's ready to walk out the door with you.

Per serving: 360 calories, 17 g protein, 60 g carbohydrates, 7 g fiber, 48 g total sugar, 7 g fat, 2 g saturated fat, 212 mg sodium, 1346 mg potassium (29% DV), 569 mg calcium (57% DV), 96 mg magnesium (24% DV), 1.37 mcg B12 (23% DV), 0.41 mg B6 (20% DV), mg iron 0.9 (5% DV)

# Eggs Florentine

    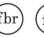 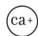

This crave-worthy brunch staple is made lighter with a few healthy substitutions and is packed with potassium and magnesium from the spinach to help combat cramps. Nutrition is boosted with whole wheat English muffins and extra spinach while the usually enormous calorie count is trimmed by using turkey bacon and a creamy and delicious faux hollandaise sauce.

makes 2 servings / prep time: 10 minutes / total time: 20 minutes

**Faux Hollandaise Sauce**

2 tablespoons 2% plain Greek yogurt

2 teaspoons freshly squeezed lemon juice

2 teaspoons melted butter

½ teaspoon Dijon mustard

¼ teaspoon garlic powder

¼ teaspoon kosher salt

1 tablespoon white vinegar

4 large eggs

2 slices turkey bacon

4 teaspoons butter

6 cups baby spinach

¼ teaspoon freshly ground black pepper

2 whole wheat English muffins

2 tablespoon hummus, divided

Dash of cayenne pepper

Dash of sweet paprika

Whisk the faux hollandaise ingredients, yogurt through salt; set aside.

Bring 1½ inches of water to a simmer in a large wide-mouthed pot. Stir in the white vinegar. Crack 1 cold egg into a small bowl and lower it to the edge of the water. Slowly release the egg into the water. Repeat with the remaining eggs. Turn off the heat, cover, and let the eggs cook for 5 minutes. Remove from the water with a slotted spoon and set aside.

Cook the turkey bacon over medium heat in a nonstick skillet until crispy, about 3 minutes per side. Cut each slice into two pieces and set aside. Add the butter to the skillet and heat until bubbling, about 1 minute. Add the spinach and black pepper and sauté until wilted, about 1 minute more.

Toast the English muffins. Spread each half with hummus, layer on spinach and a piece of bacon, then top with a poached egg and a dollop of sauce. Sprinkle each half with cayenne and paprika.

Per serving: 484 calories, 27 g protein, 36 g carbohydrates, 7 g fiber, 7 g total sugar, 27 g fat, 12 g saturated fat, 760 mg sodium, 868 mg potassium (25% DV), 348 mg calcium (35% DV), 139 mg magnesium (35% DV), 1 mcg B12 (16% DV), 0.6 mg B6 (28% DV), 6 mg iron (35% DV)

Healthy, Happy Pregnancy Cookbook

# Cramp Destroying Kale Salad with Avocado, Strawberries, Edamame, and Goat Cheese

This salad is refreshing, bursting with flavor, and packed with potassium to help prevent pesky muscle cramping. Massaging the kale helps break down its fibers and softens it to an almost cooked texture. The salad is also a complete meal, offering up protein from the edamame and healthy carbohydrate from quinoa.

makes 4 servings / prep time: 15 minutes / total time: 15 minutes

**Dressing**

**3 tablespoons extra-virgin olive oil**

**2 tablespoons white wine vinegar**

**Finely grated zest of 1 Meyer lemon**

**2 tablespoons freshly squeezed Meyer lemon juice**

**½ garlic clove, minced**

**¼ teaspoon kosher salt**

**6 cups finely chopped kale leaves**

**1 avocado, cut into cubes**

**1 cup cooked quinoa**

**1 cup chopped strawberries**

**1 cup cooked shelled edamame**

**1 cup crumbled goat cheese**

In a small bowl, whisk the dressing ingredients, or shake them together in a container with a lid.

Add the kale to a large salad bowl. Pour half the dressing into the bowl with the kale. Using your hands, massage the dressing into the kale until the kale leaves are coated and have softened. Add the remaining salad ingredients and toss to combine, drizzling with the additional dressing.

Per serving: 450 calories, 20 g protein, 33 g carbohydrates, 8 g fiber, 7 g total sugar, 29 g fat, 10 g saturated fat, 261 mg sodium, 1009 mg potassium (29% DV), 351 mg calcium (35% DV), 129 mg magnesium (32% DV), 0.1 mcg B12 (1% DV), 0.5 mg B6 (26% DV), 2.2 mg iron (12% DV)

> Some women wonder about whether it's safe to have honey during pregnancy. Yes, you CAN have honey during pregnancy and breast-feeding. However, once baby comes he or she should not consume honey until the age of 1. Why? Honey may contain small amounts of a bacteria called *Clostridium botulinum*, which could cause infant botulism due to baby's immature digestive tract.

# Waldorf Chicken Salad with Pistachios and Creamy Yogurt Dressing

This dish is a healthy and delicious take on a popular chicken salad with fruit and nuts. Yogurt is used in place of half of the mayo, reducing the fat and calories and adding more protein and calcium. Pistachios offer crunch, as well as magnesium for keeping cramps away.

---

makes 4 servings / prep time: 15 minutes / total time: 30 minutes

---

1 pound boneless, skinless chicken breasts, or 2 cups chopped or shredded cooked chicken

3 cups low-sodium chicken broth

1 celery stalk with leaves, cut in half or quarters, plus ½ cup chopped celery

⅓ cup chopped apple

½ cup halved red grapes

⅓ cup pistachios, chopped


Dressing

½ cup 2% plain Greek yogurt

1½ tablespoons real mayonnaise

1 tablespoon freshly squeezed lemon juice

1 teaspoon Dijon mustard

¼ teaspoon kosher salt

¼ teaspoon freshly ground black pepper

Combine the chicken, broth, and celery stalk (but not the chopped celery) in a medium pot; the broth should cover the chicken by at least 1 inch. Bring the broth to a boil, then reduce the heat to medium-low and simmer until the chicken is cooked to an internal temperate of 165°F, about 15 minutes. Let cool, then cut the chicken into small square chunks and transfer to a salad bowl. Add the chopped celery, apple, grapes, and pistachios and toss to combine.

In a small bowl, combine the yogurt, mayonnaise, lemon juice, mustard, salt, and pepper, and mix well until creamy. Incorporate the dressing into the chicken mixture, tossing to coat.

Serve the chicken salad in whole wheat pita, on two slices of whole wheat bread, in a whole grain wrap, or over salad greens with a side of whole grain crackers.

Per serving: 374 calories, 33 g protein, 14 g carbohydrates, 2 g fiber, 8 g total sugar, 21 g fat, 5 g saturated fat, 317 mg sodium, 651 mg potassium (19% DV), 75 mg calcium (7% DV), 49 mg magnesium (12% DV), 0.6 mcg B12 (10% DV), 0.8 mg B6 (42% DV), 3.6 mg iron (20% DV)

Healthy, Happy Pregnancy Cookbook

# Twice-Baked Avocado Potatoes

A mixture of avocado and Greek yogurt creates a creamy and rich center for these cheese-topped baked potatoes. You're getting potassium from the potatoes, calcium from the cheese, and healthy fats from the avocado—cramps be gone! Serve them with a lean protein and a green salad for a complete meal.

makes 4 servings / prep time: 15 minutes / total time: 1 hour 35 minutes

2 large russet potatoes

2 teaspoons olive oil

1 ripe avocado

3 tablespoons 2% plain Greek yogurt

¼ teaspoon kosher salt

¼ teaspoon freshly ground black pepper

½ cup chopped tomatoes

4 tablespoons chopped scallions, divided

½ cup shredded light Mexican blend cheese

Preheat the oven to 350°F. Line a baking sheet with aluminum foil.

Rub each potato with 1 teaspoon of the oil. Poke fairly deep holes in the potato skin with a fork. Place the potatoes directly on the oven rack and bake for 60 minutes, or until the skin is crispy and the potato flesh feels soft. Once the potatoes are cool enough to handle, cut in half lengthwise. Using a spoon, gently scoop out the potato flesh into a medium bowl, leaving about ¼ inch of potato at the bottom of each shell.

Add the avocado, yogurt, salt, and pepper to the potato flesh and stir to combine. Using a potato masher or a fork, mash the mixture thoroughly. Gently stir in the tomatoes and 3 tablespoons of the scallions. Place the empty potato skins on the lined baking sheet. Fill the potato skins with the mashed avocado-potato mixture. Sprinkle the cheese evenly over each half. Bake for 15 minutes, or until the cheese is bubbling and browned at the edges. Serve topped with the remaining 1 tablespoon scallions.

Per serving: 253 calories, 8 g protein, 38 g carbohydrates, 5 g fiber, 3 g total sugar, 9 g fat, 2 g saturated fat, 141 mg sodium, 1007 mg potassium (29% DV), 125 mg calcium (12% DV), 58 mg magnesium (15% DV), 0.1 mcg B12 (2% DV), 0.8 mg B6 (38% DV), 1.8 mg iron (10% DV)

# Shakshuka with Chickpeas and Feta

   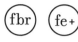  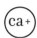

A Middle Eastern and North African dish in origin, shakshuka is one of our favorite meals and also happens to be one of the simplest comfort foods to prepare at home. Eggs are baked in a sauce of tomatoes, veggies, and spices. Tomatoes are a good source of cramp-preventing potassium, while eggs provide protein and choline for baby's brain. Eat it for breakfast, lunch, or dinner, but always serve it with warm, crusty bread or whole wheat pita that can be dipped into the sauce. A green salad rounds out the meal nicely, but it's a balanced meal on its own, too.

makes 4 servings / prep time: 10 Minutes / total time: 40 Minutes

1 tablespoon olive oil

½ yellow onion, sliced into half-moons

1 medium green bell pepper, sliced

3 garlic cloves, minced

1 (28-ounce) can whole peeled tomatoes (such as San Marzano)

2 tablespoons tomato paste

1 (14.5-ounce) can chickpeas, rinsed and drained

1 teaspoon chili powder

1 teaspoon ground cumin

1 teaspoon sweet paprika

½ teaspoon kosher salt

¼ teaspoon freshly ground black pepper, plus more for finishing

Pinch of red pepper flakes (optional)

8 large eggs

⅓ cup feta cheese

2 tablespoons chopped fresh flat-leaf parsley (optional for garnish)

Preheat the oven to 375°F.

Heat the oil in a large, deep, ovenproof skillet over medium heat. Sauté the onion and bell pepper until they soften and the onion turns slightly golden, about 10 minutes. Add the garlic and continue to sauté until fragrant, about 2 minutes more.

Add the tomatoes and tomato paste and stir until combined. Crush the tomatoes with a potato masher or fork, leaving some chunks. Add the chickpeas, chili powder, cumin, paprika, salt, black pepper, and red pepper flakes and stir well. Simmer over medium heat for 7 to 8 minutes, or until the sauce has reduced by one-third.

Make eight evenly spaced indentations in the sauce. Crack the eggs, one at a time, directly into the indentations. Transfer the skillet to the oven and bake for 20 minutes, or until the egg whites are opaque and yolks are cooked through, adding feta over the top during the last 5 minutes of cooking. Garnish with the parsley, if using, and season with black pepper.

Per serving: 386 calories, 23 g protein, 35 g carbohydrates, 7 g fiber, 9 g total sugar, 17 g fat, 6 g saturated fat, 779 mg sodium, 358 mg potassium (10% DV), 255 mg calcium (25% DV), 28 mg magnesium (7% DV), 1 mcg B12 (18% DV), 0.4 mg B6 (19% DV), 4.2 mg iron (23% DV)

Did you know that most feta (and other soft cheeses such as goat and Brie) that you can purchase at the grocery store is pasteurized? And that the only reason to avoid any soft cheeses is to avoid eating unpasteurized cheese? In other words, you CAN eat feta cheese, just make sure you read the label first. It should say "pasteurized milk" on the ingredients label.

# Corn Farroto with Seared Scallops

If you love creamy risotto, you will love this recipe. It highlights farro, a whole grain form of wheat that has more fiber and nutrients than traditional arborio risotto rice, but cooks up with a similar texture. It's a perfect summer dish using fresh corn and basil, but you can also substitute frozen corn if you're making it in the winter and it will still taste delicious. The scallops are rich in iron, protein, potassium, and magnesium so you'll be fighting cramps while enjoying this yummy satisfying dinner.

makes 4 servings / prep time: 10 minutes / total time: 40 minutes

- 2 tablespoons olive oil, divided
- ¾ cup chopped onion
- 2 teaspoons garlic, minced
- 1¼ cups uncooked farro (regular or semi-pearled)
- ½ teaspoon kosher salt, divided
- 4 cups chicken broth, divided
- 1 tablespoon freshly squeezed lemon juice
- 1 pound sea scallops
- ¼ cup balsamic vinegar
- Freshly ground black pepper
- 1 cup cooked fresh corn kernals (about 1 large ear), or frozen and thawed
- ⅓ cup grated Parmesan cheese
- 3 tablespoons chopped fresh basil, divided
- 1 teaspoon unsalted butter

Heat 1½ tablespoons of the oil over medium heat in a 3- to 3½-quart pot. Add the onion and cook until soft, about 5 minutes. Add the garlic, and cook until fragrant, about 1 minute longer. Add the farro and ¼ teaspoon of the salt, stirring to coat the farro in the oil. Cook until the farro begins to crackle, about 2 minutes, stirring constantly. Stir in 1 cup of the broth and the lemon juice, and cook, stirring, until the liquid has been absorbed, about 5 minutes. Add 2 cups of the broth and bring to a boil. Reduce to a simmer, cover, and cook until the farro is tender, about 30 minutes. (If you're cooking semi-pearled farro, the cooking time will be closer to 15 to 20 minutes.) Stir the farro intermittently throughout the cooking time, making sure there is some liquid in the pot. If all the liquid has been absorbed before the farro is tender, add the additional broth, in ½-cup increments.

While the farro is cooking, pat the scallops dry with a paper towel and season with the remaining ¼ teaspoon salt and the black pepper to taste.

Heat the remaining ½ tablespoon oil in a medium skillet over medium-high heat. Once the oil is hot, add the scallops, spacing them evenly in the pan, and cook until browned on each side and cooked through, about 1½ minutes per side. Remove the scallops from the pan and set aside, covering loosely with foil to keep them warm.

Reduce the heat to medium. In the same skillet, add the vinegar and ¼ cup of the remaining broth and bring to a boil. Then reduce the heat to medium and cook, stirring continuously, until it thickens, 1 to 2 minutes.

Once the farro is tender, stir in the corn, Parmesan, 2 tablespoons of the basil, and the butter. Serve the farro warm, topped with the scallops, and garnished with the remaining 1 tablespoon basil.

Per serving: 445 calories, 34 g protein, 76 g carbohydrates, 12 g fiber, 7 g total sugar, 14 g fat, 3 g saturated fat, 795 mg sodium, 751 mg potassium (16% DV), 128 mg calcium (13% DV), 65 mg magnesium (16% DV), 2.02 mcg B12 (84% DV), 0.264 mg B6 (20% DV), 4 mg iron (15%)

# Cashew-Crusted Pork Tenderloin with Apples and Fennel

Apples, fennel, and a flavorful cashew crust keeps this lean cut of pork moist and flavorful. To keep away cramps, this dish provides an excellent source of magnesium and potassium, in addition to being high in iron to keep your energy up.

makes 4 servings / prep time: 15 minutes / total time: 45 minutes

1¼ pounds pork tenderloin roast

½ teaspoon kosher salt

½ teaspoon freshly ground black pepper

3 teaspoons olive oil, divided

¼ cup cashews halves

¼ cup panko bread crumbs

1 tablespoon coarsely chopped fresh flat-leaf parsley

2 teaspoons chopped garlic

1 teaspoon fennel seeds

¼ teaspoon sweet paprika

¼ cup water

1 apple, cored and cut into medium slices (about ¼ inch thick)

1 bulb fennel, trimmed and cut into slices (about ¼ inch thick)

Preheat the oven to 400°F.

Pat the tenderloin roast dry with a paper towel and sprinkle with the salt and pepper. Brush 1 teaspoon of the oil onto all sides of the pork. Set aside.

In a food processor or blender, add the cashews, bread crumbs, parsley, garlic, fennel seeds, and paprika. Pulse until the mixture is combined into coarse crumbs, but before it's a fine powder or paste. Cover all sides of the tenderloin in the cashew crust, pressing it on to help the mixture adhere to the meat.

Pour about ¼ cup water in the bottom of a 9 x 13-inch baking dish or roasting pan. Add the pork roast to the pan. Toss the apple and fennel slices with the remaining 2 teaspoons oil and arrange the slices around the pork roast in the pan.

Roast until the pork reaches an internal temperature of 145°F, 25 to 30 minutes. Let the meat rest for at least 5 minutes before slicing.

Per serving: 298 calories, 33 g protein, 18 g carbohydrates, 4 g fiber, 5 g total sugar, 11 g fat, 2 g saturated fat, 283 mg sodium, 936 mg potassium (20% DV), 55 mg calcium (6% DV), 78   mg magnesium (20% DV), 0.7 mcg B12 (30% DV), 1.1 mg B6 (92% DV), 2.7 mg iron (15% DV)

# Seasoned Carrot Fries

Carrots are cut into fry-size sticks and roasted in olive oil until slightly crispy. These are so delicious you'll probably want to make a double batch. And not to get ahead of things, but they're great for when baby starts eating solids, too!

makes 4 servings / prep time: 5 minutes / total time: 25 minutes

**8 medium carrots**

**1½ tablespoons olive oil**

**¼ teaspoon garlic powder**

**¼ teaspoon sweet paprika**

**½ teaspoon kosher salt**

**½ teaspoon freshly ground black pepper**

**Ketchup, mustard, or peanut sauce, for dipping**

Preheat the oven to 400°F.

Trim the ends off the carrots and slice the carrots in half crosswise. Then cut each half, lengthwise, into ¼-inch-thick strips. Stir together the oil, garlic powder, paprika, salt, and pepper in a small bowl. Toss the carrot sticks with the olive oil–spice mixture until well coated. Spread the carrots evenly on a baking sheet, being careful not to let fries touch or overlap. Bake until golden and slightly crispy, turning once throughout baking time, about 20 minutes.

Serve with ketchup, mustard, or peanut sauce for dipping.

Per serving: 97 calories, 1 g protein, 12 g carbohydrates, 4 g fiber, 6 g total sugar, 5 g fat, <1 g saturated fat, 225 mg sodium, 400 mg potassium (11% DV), 42 mg calcium (4% DV), 16 mg magnesium (4% DV), 0 mcg B12 (0% DV), 0.2 mg B6 (9% DV), 0.3 mg iron (2% DV)

# CHAPTER SIX

# I Want Chocolate . . . with Peanuts and Pickles! Recipes to Satisfy Every Craving

So you're eating healthy to nourish you and baby throughout this nine-month (but really it's ten!) journey. But what about nourishing that little voice inside of you who's saying (screaming) must. have. comfort food. now!? We've got you covered.

In this chapter you'll find recipes for everything from chocolate and pizza to cheesesteaks and mashed potatoes. Oh, and pickles. They're in here, too.

We've heard about, and experienced, all kinds of strange cravings during pregnancy. We don't claim to cover every combination you can dream up, but we certainly cover the standard cravings. That's what these recipes are all about. And, since you've got to fit the foods you crave into an overall healthy diet, without TOO many added calories (those extra 300 calories you need can be gobbled up faster than you can say three-quarters cup Ben & Jerry's), these recipes will satisfy your cravings without putting you over the top. In addition, they'll even add valuable nutrients like healthy fats, B vitamins, calcium, and iron.

# Peanut Butter, Apple, and Chickpea Breakfast Cookies

Cookies for breakfast? This is something we can get on board with, and bet you can, too. This flourless cookie contains all the makings of a healthy breakfast in a cookie form you'll crave with a glass of milk! The chickpeas lend a healthy dose of fiber, while chia seeds deliver protein and nutritious omega-3 fats. Both are essential building blocks for baby. Nosh two with a glass of milk (or calcium-fortified alternative) for a healthy breakfast.

makes 6 servings (2 cookies per serving) / prep time: 10 minutes / total time: 22 minutes

**1 (15-ounce) can chickpeas, rinsed, drained, and blotted with a paper towel or kitchen towel**

**½ cup salted natural peanut butter**

**⅓ cup maple syrup**

**1 teaspoon baking powder**

**1 tablespoon chia seeds**

**2 teaspoons pure vanilla extract**

**½ cup finely chopped apples**

Preheat the oven to 350°F.

Combine the chickpeas, peanut butter, maple syrup, baking powder, chia seeds, and vanilla in a food processor or high-powered blender. Blend until smooth, scraping down the sides as needed, about 30 seconds. Transfer the dough to a bowl.

Fold in the chopped apples. Form the dough into 12 equal balls, then flatten each slightly with the back of a fork or spoon. Place the cookies on a baking sheet, spacing them at least 1 inch apart. Bake for 12 to 14 minutes, or until the outsides are golden and firm. The insides will still be slightly softer than a regular cookie. Store cooled cookies in an airtight container for up to 5 days.

Per serving: 126 calories, 5 g protein, 13 g carbohydrates, 2 g fiber, 5 g total sugar, 7 g fat, <1 g saturated fat, 46 mg sodium, 86 mg potassium (2% DV), 7 mg magnesium (2% DV), 0 mcg B12 (0% DV), .001 mg B6 (0% DV), 0.6 mg iron (4% DV)

# Crispy French Toast Fingers with Creamy Strawberry-Chia Dipping Sauce

If you're craving something sweet to begin your day, skip the sugary stuff you'll find at your local diner and opt for this version. The chia seeds add extra protein and fiber, something most French toast is lacking.

makes 2 servings / prep time: 10 minutes / total time: 20 minutes

2 large eggs

3 tablespoons 2% plain Greek yogurt, divided

1 tablespoon maple syrup

1 teaspoon pure vanilla extract

½ teaspoon ground cinnamon

1½ cups crushed whole grain flake cereal (such as Nature's Path Heritage Flakes)

3 slices 2- to 3-day-old whole wheat bread (⅓- to ½-inch-thick slices)

1 tablespoon coconut oil or unsalted butter

1 cup frozen strawberries

1 teaspoon orange zest

¼ cup orange juice

¼ cup water

1 tablespoon chia seeds

Whisk the eggs, 2 tablespoons of the yogurt, the maple syrup, vanilla, and cinnamon in a shallow bowl. Fill a separate shallow bowl with the cereal flakes. Dip both sides of each bread slice in the egg batter. Then dip both sides of each slice of bread into the cereal flakes, pressing gently to coat.

Heat the oil in a medium skillet over medium-high heat. Add the coated bread slices to the skillet and cook until golden and crispy, about 3 minutes per side.

Meanwhile, in a small saucepan over medium heat, combine the strawberries, orange zest, orange juice, and water and bring to a boil. Reduce to a simmer, add the chia seeds, and cook for 10 minutes, mashing the strawberries with a fork or pureeing with an immersion blender while cooking. Turn off the heat, let sit an additional 10 minutes, then stir in the remaining 1 tablespoon yogurt.

Cut the French toast into 1-inch strips, divide between 2 plates, and dip into the sauce.

Per serving: 402 calories, 16 g protein, 56 g carbohydrates, 8 g fiber, 32 g total sugar, 14 g fat, 6 g saturated fat, 284 mg sodium, 496 mg potassium (14% DV), 195 mg calcium (19% DV) 87 mg magnesium (22% DV), 0.5 mcg B12 (7% DV), 0.2 mg B6 (13% DV), 1.4 mg iron (7% DV)

# Sun-Dried Tomato, Swiss Chard, and Feta Quiche with Oat-Almond Crust

Quiche is typically a high-calorie, rich meal made with heavy cream and nestled in a butter-laden crust. This version is just as delicious, but incorporates ingredients that add nutrition and lighten the dish up a bit. It starts with a nutty oat and almond crust, and is filled with an egg mixture that contains protein-rich cottage cheese that also delivers a creamy texture. Swiss chard stands up perfectly to the eggs and is packed with beta-carotene, vitamin C, and iron, important nutrients for your growing little human. Pair a slice with a piece of fresh fruit for a complete breakfast.

makes 6 servings / prep time: 15 minutes + 1 hour refrigeration / total time: 1 hour 10 minutes + 1 hour refrigeration

### Crust

1 cup old-fashioned rolled oats

⅓ cup almond meal or almond flour

¼ teaspoon sea salt

3 tablespoons cold unsalted butter, cut into small pieces

3 tablespoons cold buttermilk

### Filling

1 teaspoon olive oil

½ cup chopped onion

4 cups chopped Swiss chard, stems and leaves separated

½ teaspoon salt

½ cup chopped sun-dried tomatoes

4 large whole eggs

2 large egg whites

1 cup 1% milk

½ cup low-fat cottage cheese

½ cup crumbled feta cheese

To prepare the crust, combine the oats, almond meal, and salt in a food processor and process until the ingredients are combined and oats are ground into small pieces. Add the butter and pulse until the mixture forms little pebbles. Slowly add the buttermilk until the dough is uniform. Remove the dough and form into a flat disk. Place the disk between two layers of wax or parchment pepper. Refrigerate for 1 hour, or up to 2 days.

When you're ready to assemble and bake the quiche, preheat the oven to 375°F.

Roll out the dough into a 10-inch circle with the wax or parchment paper still on the bottom. Once rolled out, turn a 9-inch pie dish over it so it's upside down on top of the crust, then flip both over and press the crust into the dish, using the paper to help.

Healthy, Happy Pregnancy Cookbook

If it breaks apart anywhere just press it back together. Par-bake the crust until it turns golden, 5 to 7 minutes, then set aside to cool. Reduce the oven temperature to 350°F.

Meanwhile, heat the oil in a medium skillet over medium-high heat. Reduce the heat to medium, add the onion, and sauté for 5 minutes, or until translucent and beginning soften. Add the chard stems and sauté until tender, another 5 minutes. Add the chard leaves and the salt, sauté until wilted and softened, about 5 minutes more. Stir in the sun-dried tomatoes and sprinkle this mixture evenly over the bottom of the pre-baked crust.

In a large bowl, whisk together the eggs, egg whites, milk, and cottage cheese. Pour the custard over the veggies in the pie dish. Sprinkle the feta cheese evenly over the top.

Bake the quiche until the eggs are set and the top has turned slightly golden, 40 to 45 minutes. Let cool at least 10 minutes before cutting and serving.

Per serving: 287 calories, 16 g protein, 19 g carbohydrates, 3 g fiber, 7 g total sugar, 17 g fat, 8 g saturated fat, 663 mg sodium, 475 mg potassium (14% DV), 181 mg calcium (18% DV), 80 mg magnesium (20% DV), 0.9 mcg B12 (15% DV), 0.2 mg B6 (10% DV), 2.4 mg iron (13% DV)

# Panko-Coconut Chicken Tenders with Honey-Mustard Dipping Sauce

Panko bread crumbs and shredded coconut make the perfect crispy coating to these baked chicken tenders, which will likely become a staple in your meal rotation. They deliver the satisfaction and flavor of fried chicken tenders, but without the heaviness of deep-frying.

makes 6 servings / prep time: 15 minutes / total time: 30 minutes

¼ cup whole wheat flour

1 large egg, lightly beaten

2 teaspoons Dijon mustard

1 cup panko bread crumbs

½ cup unsweetened coconut flakes

½ teaspoon freshly ground black pepper

½ teaspoon kosher salt

1¼ pounds chicken breast tenders

Cooking spray

Dipping Sauce

3 tablespoons low-fat plain Greek yogurt

1 tablespoon honey

1 tablespoon Dijon mustard

½ teaspoon dried rosemary

Preheat the oven to 425°F.

Fill a wide, shallow bowl with the flour. In a separate shallow bowl, whisk together the egg and mustard. Fill a third shallow bowl with the bread crumbs, coconut, pepper, and salt.

Dredge the chicken in the flour until each piece has a light, even coating. Dip the floured chicken into the egg mixture, shaking off the excess, and then dip into the bread crumb mixture, lightly pressing the chicken into the crumbs to coat evenly. Spray each side of the tenders with cooking spray.

Place the tenders on a wire rack set over a baking sheet. Bake the chicken until browned and crispy and cooked to an internal temperature of 165°F, about 15 minutes.

Stir together the yogurt, honey, mustard, and rosemary until smooth and serve as a dipping sauce.

Per serving: 263 calories, 25 g protein, 22 g carbohydrates, 3 g fiber, 4 g total sugar, 8.5 g fat, 5 g saturated fat, 360 mg sodium, 405 mg potassium (% DV), 30 mg calcium (3% DV), 41 mg magnesium (0% DV), 0.263 mcg B12 (0% DV), 0.766 mg B6 (0% DV), 1.3 mg iron (7% DV)

# Classic Tomato-Basil Marinara Sauce

You don't have to spend hours at the stove to make a delicious homemade marinara. This recipe is well worth the 30 minutes, most of which are spent listening for the timer to indicate your restaurant-worthy sauce is ready. The simple-but-flavorful ingredients will make a difference in your next Italian recipe. Or, simply serve this marinara over a bed of whole wheat pasta tossed with wilted greens and top with a flourish of Parmesan cheese. This sauce is also perfect for freezing, so you always have a great marinara on hand.

makes 4 servings (about 2 ½ cups) / prep time: 5 minutes / total time: 30 minutes

1 (28-ounce) can good-quality whole peeled tomatoes (such as San Marzano)

14 ounces water

2 tablespoons olive oil

1 cup diced yellow onion

4 garlic cloves, thinly sliced

½ teaspoon kosher salt

½ teaspoon freshly ground black pepper

¼ teaspoon dried oregano

¼ teaspoon red pepper flakes

½ cup whole fresh basil leaves

Add the tomatoes and the water to a large bowl. Using a potato masher or your hands, gently crush the tomatoes. Set aside.

Heat the oil in a large, deep skillet or saucepot over medium heat. Add the onion and cook until soft and sweet, about 12 minutes. Add the garlic, salt, black pepper, oregano, red pepper flakes, and basil. Stir to combine and cook until the garlic is fragrant, about 1 minute.

Add the tomatoes and let simmer vigorously until the sauce thickens, about 25 minutes. For a smoother sauce, blend the sauce in the skillet with a handheld immersion blender, leaving some textured and some smooth.

Per serving: 87 calories, 2 g protein, 10 g carbohydrates, 2 g fiber, 4 g total sugar, 5 g fat, <1 g saturated fat, 303 mg sodium, 56 mg potassium (2% DV), 59 mg calcium (6% DV), 5 mg magnesium (1% DV), 0 mcg B12 (0% DV), 0.1 mg B6 (3% DV), 0.5 mg iron (3% DV)

# Baked Panko Eggplant Parmesan

  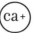

Craving warm, ooey-gooey, cheesy comfort food? In this classic Italian dish, panko bread crumbs add a crisp shell to the eggplant that replaces frying. Consider making two and freezing one for later.

makes 4 servings / prep time: 15 minutes / total time: 1 hour 15 minutes

1 teaspoon olive oil

1 large whole egg

1 large egg white

1½ cups panko bread crumbs

¼ teaspoon dried oregano

¼ teaspoon kosher salt

1 large eggplant, sliced crosswise into ¼-inch, round slices (you need at least 12 slices)

2 cups marinara sauce (store-bought or see recipe on page 127)

2 cups chopped baby spinach, divided

¾ cup shredded part-skim mozzarella cheese, divided

½ cup grated Parmesan cheese, divided

⅓ cup coarsely chopped fresh basil, divided

Preheat the oven to 375°F. Grease a large baking sheet with the oil.

Whisk the whole egg with the egg white in a shallow bowl until frothy. In a separate shallow bowl, combine the bread crumbs, oregano, and salt and stir to combine. Dip both sides of each eggplant in the egg wash, then coat with the bread crumbs and place on the baking sheet.

Bake the eggplant until each slice is soft and the bread crumbs have begun to brown, flipping once halfway through, about 20 minutes.

When the eggplant has finished cooking, turn the oven up to 400°F. Spread one-third of the marinara on the bottom of a 13 x 9-inch or 11 x 7-inch baking dish. Add a layer of 6 baked eggplant rounds. Top with another one-third of the sauce, half the spinach, half the mozzarella, half the Parmesan, and half the basil. Repeat with the next layer of eggplant, the remaining sauce, the remaining spinach, and the remaining mozzarella and Parmesan. Finish by sprinkling with the remaining basil. Bake until the cheeses begin to brown and bubble, about 20 minutes.

Per serving: 356 calories, 19 g protein, 38 g carbohydrates, 8 g fiber, 10 g total sugar, 15 g fat, 6 g saturated fat, 752 mg sodium, 533 mg potassium (11% DV), 395 mg calcium (40% DV) 51 mg magnesium (13% DV), 0.9 mcg B12 (37% DV), 0.256 mg B6 (20% DV), 2.5 mg iron (14% DV)

Healthy, Happy Pregnancy Cookbook

# Chicken Sausage Pizza on Whole Wheat Pizza Crust

This semi-homemade pizza will crush your cravings, but is packed with way more nutrition than delivery! It feels decadent thanks to the sausage and cheese, but is much lower in saturated fat, sodium, and calories, and provides a good dose of fiber and veggies.

makes 4 servings / prep time: 10 minutes / total time: 35 minutes

1 tablespoon olive oil

1 medium yellow onion, sliced in half-moons

16 ounces refrigerated whole wheat pizza dough (find in the deli section of your store, the frozen aisle, or ask at the bakery if they make it fresh), at room temperature

2 pre-cooked sweet Italian chicken sausages, chopped

1½ cups chopped baby spinach leaves

⅔ cup marinara sauce (store-bought or see recipe on page 127)

¾ cup shredded part-skim mozzarella cheese

Preheat the oven to 425°F. Heat the oil in a medium skillet over medium heat. Add the onion and cook until it begins to turn a caramel color, turning down the heat if the onion begins to burn, about 15 minutes.

While the onion cooks, work the pizza dough into a 12-inch circle (or rectangle) on a floured surface. Poke a few holes in the crust with a fork to prevent large bubbles from forming during baking. Transfer the dough onto a pizza stone or a lightly oiled baking sheet. Par-bake the crust for 5 minutes.

Add the sausage to the onion and cook until the sausage begins to brown, 3 to 4 minutes more. Add the spinach and sauté until just wilted, about 1 minute. Turn off the heat.

Spread the marinara over the crust. Top with the onion mixture and sprinkle with the mozzarella. Bake until the dough is slightly browned at the edges and cheese is bubbling, about 10 minutes.

Per serving: 429 calories, 23 g protein, 54 g carbohydrates, 9 g fiber, 5 g total sugar, 15 g fat, 4 g saturated fat, 787 mg sodium, 802 mg potassium (23% DV), 226 mg calcium (23% DV), 18 mg magnesium (5% DV), 0.5 mcg B12 (20% DV), 0.08 mg B6 (7% DV), 2.6 mg iron (14% DV)

# Baked Mac and Cheese with Roasted Cauliflower

This creamy comfort dish gets a flavor and nutrition boost from roasted cauliflower. It's half pasta and half cauliflower, which makes the dish more interesting from a texture and flavor standpoint, and saves calories and saturated fat in the process. Using Greek yogurt and low-fat milk in place of a traditional roux also helps cut back on calories and extra saturated fat.

makes 6 servings / prep time: 10 minutes / total time: 40 minutes

1 medium head cauliflower, cored and coarsely chopped (about 3 cups)

2½ tablespoons olive oil, divided

10 ounces uncooked whole wheat rotini (about 2½ cups)

⅓ cup whole wheat bread crumbs

½ cup fresh flat-leaf parsley

1 teaspoon salt, divided

½ teaspoon freshly ground black pepper, divided

½ cup chopped onion

1½ cups grated extra-sharp cheddar cheese

½ cup grated Parmesan cheese

1 cup 2% plain Greek yogurt

½ cup 1% milk

½ teaspoon mustard powder

¼ teaspoon garlic powder

¼ teaspoon paprika

Preheat the oven to 400°F. Line a baking sheet with aluminum foil.

Toss the cauliflower with 1 tablespoon of the oil and bake on the baking sheet until the cauliflower begins to brown on the edges and is soft, about 15 minutes.

Cook the pasta according to the package directions. While the pasta is cooking, pulse the bread crumbs in a food processor or blender together with the parsley, 1 tablespoon of the oil, ¼ teaspoon of the salt, and ¼ teaspoon of the pepper. Set aside.

Drain the pasta. Return the empty pasta pot to medium heat and add the remaining ½ tablespoon oil. Add the onion and the remaining ¾ teaspoon salt, and the remaining ¼ teaspoon pepper and cook, stirring occasionally, until the onion is soft, 3 to 5 minutes.

Mix in the pasta, cauliflower, cheddar, Parmesan, yogurt, milk, mustard powder, garlic powder, and paprika. Stir to combine all the ingredients. Transfer to a shallow 3-quart baking dish, sprinkle with the bread crumb mixture, and bake until golden brown, 12 to 15 minutes.

Per serving: 316 calories, 19 g protein, 23 g carbohydrates, 4 g fiber, 7 g total sugar, 18 g fat, 9 g saturated fat, 520 mg sodium, 410 mg potassium (9% DV), 402 mg calcium (40% DV) 48 mg magnesium (12% DV), 0.5 mcg B12 (20% DV), 0.264 mg B6 (20% DV), 1.5 mg iron (8% DV)

Healthy, Happy Pregnancy Cookbook

# Chicken and Pinto Bean Nachos

A little surprised that nachos can stand alone as a healthy meal? These nachos are just as delicious as the ones you'll get at your local Mexican or fast casual restaurant, but they're packed with lots of nutrition for half the calories. The key is loading them with veggies and fiber- and protein-rich beans, and using smaller but flavorful portions of higher-calorie ingredients like cheese and sour cream (which we've substituted with Greek yogurt).

makes 4 servings / prep time: 10 minutes / total time: 25 minutes

4 ounces corn tortilla chips

2 teaspoons olive oil

½ cup chopped yellow onion

1 cup chopped baby spinach

1 (15-ounce) can pinto beans, rinsed and drained

¼ cup salsa

½ teaspoon ground cumin

¼ teaspoon garlic powder

1 cup shredded cooked skinless chicken breast

1 cup shredded sharp cheddar cheese

1 jalapeño pepper, seeds removed, sliced into thin rings

1 cup chopped tomatoes

¼ cup sliced scallions

¼ cup 2% plain Greek yogurt

Preheat the oven to 350°F. Arrange the tortilla chips on an aluminum foil–lined baking sheet or in a 2- to 2½-quart casserole dish.

In a medium skillet over medium-high heat, heat the oil. Add the onion and cook until softened, stirring occasionally, about 7 minutes. Reduce the heat to medium-low. Add the spinach, beans, salsa, cumin, and garlic powder and stir to combine. Mash the beans slightly with a fork or potato masher until some are mashed and some are still whole. Remove the skillet from the heat.

Top the tortilla chips evenly with the bean mixture. Layer on the shredded chicken, cheese, jalapeño, and tomatoes. Bake the nachos for 10 to 15 minutes, or until the cheese is bubbly. Sprinkle with the scallions and top each serving with a dollop of yogurt.

Per serving: 450 calories, 27 g protein, 40 g carbohydrates, 7 g fiber, 5 g total sugar, 21 g fat, 8 g saturated fat, 809 mg sodium, 248 mg potassium (7% DV), 33 mg calcium (3% DV), 31 mg magnesium (8% DV), 0.35 mcg B12 (15% DV), 0.40 mg B6 (32% DV), 2.6 mg iron (14% DV)

# Cheddar "Philly" Cheesesteak Wrap

Using a lean cut of beef and flavorful sharp cheddar cheese, along with lower-fat milk in place of heavy cream and butter in the sauce, allows this recipe to taste rich while still delivering nutrients but not excessive calories. It's also packed with onions and peppers so you get your veggies all in one.

makes 2 servings / prep time: 10 minutes / total time: 25 minutes

**6 ounces top loin steak, chilled in the freezer for 15 minutes prior to cooking**

**¼ teaspoon kosher salt**

**½ teaspoon freshly ground black pepper**

**¼ teaspoon garlic powder**

**4 teaspoons olive oil, divided**

**½ medium yellow onion, sliced into half-moons**

**1 large red bell pepper, sliced**

**2 (8- to 10-inch) whole wheat tortillas, warmed**

**1 cup chopped romaine lettuce (optional)**

Cheese Sauce

**⅓ cup 1% milk or unsweetened dairy-free alternative**

**2 teaspoons all-purpose flour**

**½ cup shredded extra-sharp cheddar cheese**

Slicing against the grain, cut the beef into thin (¼-inch) strips. Sprinkle the beef with the salt, black pepper, and garlic powder. Heat 2 teaspoons of the oil in a large skillet over medium-high heat. Add the steak and sauté until browned and just cooked through, about 5 minutes. Set aside.

Heat the remaining 2 teaspoons oil in the skillet. Add the onion and bell pepper and toss to coat in the oil. Reduce the heat to medium and cook until the vegetables are soft and the onion has begun to turn a caramel color, 12 to 15 minutes.

Make the cheese sauce by whisking the milk and flour in a small saucepan until the flour is fully incorporated. Turn the heat to medium-high and continue to stir until thickened, about 2 minutes. Stir in the cheese and continue to stir until creamy, adding warm water if necessary to thin it out, 2 to 3 minutes longer.

Once the vegetables have finished cooking, add the steak back to the skillet and cook until everything is hot, about 1 minute.

Divide the steak and bell peppers evenly over the center of each tortilla and pour the cheese sauce over the top. Add the lettuce, if desired. Roll each tortilla to close.

Per serving: 569 calories, 32 g protein, 42 g carbohydrates, 6 g fiber, 7 g total sugar, 30 g fat, 12 g saturated fat, 637 mg sodium, 759 mg potassium 16% DV), 307 mg calcium (31% DV) 88 mg magnesium (22% DV), 1.3 mcg B12 (55% DV), 0.89 mg B6 (69% DV), 3.9 mg iron (22% DV)

Healthy, Happy Pregnancy Cookbook

# Cauliflower-Potato Mash with Mushroom Gravy

Traditional mashed potatoes and gravy often come with a calorie and saturated fat count that can weigh you down before you get your nutrient fill. This recipe uses a mix of cauliflower and potato to deliver potato flavor and texture with an extra serving of veggies.

makes 4 servings / prep time: 10 minutes / total time: 30 minutes

### Cauliflower-Potato Mash

- 2 medium Yukon Gold potatoes, peeled or unpeeled and quartered
- 2 cups cauliflower florets
- 1 tablespoon butter or vegan spread
- ¼ cup 1% milk or dairy-free alternative
- 2 tablespoons 2% plain Greek yogurt (optional)
- ¼ teaspoon garlic powder
- ¼ teaspoon salt
- ¼ teaspoon freshly ground black pepper, or to taste

### Mushroom Gravy

- 2 teaspoons olive oil
- 1 teaspoon butter
- 1 teaspoon minced garlic
- 1 tablespoon minced shallot
- 2 cups sliced white or cremini mushrooms
- 2 tablespoons whole wheat flour
- ½ cup low-sodium chicken or vegetable stock
- ¼ teaspoon dried thyme

Put the potatoes in a medium pot and cover with cold water. Bring to a boil, then reduce the heat to a simmer and cook until the potatoes are fork-tender, about 15 minutes. While the potatoes are cooking, place a steamer basket on top of the potato pot to steam the cauliflower, or steam the cauliflower in the microwave until tender, 3 to 4 minutes. When the potatoes and cauliflower have finished cooking, drain in a colander and set aside.

Heat the butter and milk over low heat in the pot that the potatoes were cooked in until the butter has melted and the milk is warm, about 5 minutes. Add the potatoes, cauliflower, yogurt (if using), garlic powder, salt, and pepper. Mash with a potato masher (or use an immersion blender) until you reach your desired consistency. We like to leave ours a bit chunky!

For the gravy, heat the oil and butter in a medium skillet over medium-high heat. Add the garlic and shallot and sauté until fragrant, about 1 minute. Add the mushrooms and sauté until soft, about 5 minutes. Reduce the heat to medium, stir in the flour, then cook for another 2 minutes. Stir in the stock and thyme and simmer until thickened. Serve the gravy over the mash.

Per serving: 197 calories, 7 g protein, 29 g carbohydrates, 5 g fiber, 4 g total sugar, 7 g fat, 3 g saturated fat, 255 mg sodium, 802 mg potassium (23% DV), 61 mg calcium (6% DV), 45 mg magnesium (11% DV), 0.1 mcg B12 (2% DV), 0.5 mg B6 (26% DV), 1.2 mg iron (6% DV)

# Dark Chocolate Pecan Banana Bites

Banana pieces are dipped in dark chocolate, topped with chopped pecans, and frozen to mimic the flavors and textures of favorite store-bought frozen treats. These are the perfect bites to have in the freezer when a chocolate or dessert craving hits. Before eating, set a couple pieces out at room temperature for a minute or two. The banana will soften just enough and resemble the consistency of ice cream.

makes 6 servings (12 bites total) / prep time: 20 minutes / total time: 3 hours 20 minutes (including freeze time)

**½ cup dark chocolate chunks, chips, or pieces**

**2 teaspoons coconut oil**

**2 large bananas, sliced into ½-inch chunks**

**½ cup chopped pecans**

Put the chocolate and oil in a shallow, microwave-safe bowl. Microwave on high for 30 seconds, then stir the chocolate and oil to combine. Continue to microwave and stir in 15- to 30-second increments, until smooth, 2 to 3 cycles.

Arrange the banana chunks on a plate or small baking sheet covered with parchment paper. Using a fork or a toothpick to spear the banana slices, dip each slice in the chocolate, coating the top and sides. Place the banana bites down on the parchment paper, chocolate-coated side up, then sprinkle the pecans over the top.

Freeze on the parchment paper until solid, at least 3 hours or overnight. Once frozen, transfer the bites to a sealed bag or container and store in the freezer.

Per serving: 144 calories, 6 g protein, 30 g carbohydrates, 8 g fiber, 20 g total sugar, 6 g fat, 1 g saturated fat, 371 mg sodium, 896 mg potassium (26% DV), 408 mg calcium (41% DV), 115 mg magnesium (29% DV), 0 mcg B12 (0% DV), 0.09 mg B6 (4% DV), 0.7 mg iron (4% DV)

Healthy, Happy Pregnancy Cookbook

# Cold Cocoa

This chilly drink packs a serious chocolate punch and will satisfy chocolate cravings almost instantly while also hydrating. Coconut water provides electrolytes, while maple syrup delivers just a hint of flavorful sweetness without loading you up with sugar.

makes 1 serving / prep time: 5 minutes / total time: 5 minutes

1 cup coconut water

¾ cup unsweetened almond milk or skim milk

2 tablespoons unsweetened cocoa powder

1 tablespoon maple syrup

¼ teaspoon pure vanilla extract

Handful of ice cubes

Pour the coconut water and milk into a tall glass or mason jar with a lid. Stir in the cocoa powder, maple syrup, and vanilla. Stir briskly, whisk, or shake gently until all of the cocoa powder is mixed thoroughly into the liquid and the drink is smooth, 1 to 2 minutes. If it takes longer, keep stirring until all of the cocoa is incorporated. Add the ice, and gently shake again until slightly frothy.

Per serving: 220 calories, 6 g protein, 40 g carbohydrates, 6 g fiber, 32 g total sugar, 6 g fat, 1 g saturated fat, 371 mg sodium, 770 mg potassium (22% DV), 854 mg calcium (85% DV), 142 mg magnesium (36% DV), 5 mcg B12 (85% DV), 0.09 mg B6 (4% DV), 2.8 mg iron (16% DV)

# Crunchy Chili-Cumin Chickpeas

When you're craving a crunchy, salty snack, but also want to pack some nutrition into your day, skip the pretzels and reach for the chickpeas! Chickpeas (garbanzo beans) are roasted to crunchy, golden perfection and coated with a chili spice mixture that will keep your taste buds interested. The balance of protein and fiber will give you energy without the kind of crash that follows pretzels or chips. Plus, one serving of these little guys is REALLY satisfying.

makes 4 servings / prep time: 5 minutes / total time: 35 minutes

**1 (14.5-ounce) can chickpeas**

**1 tablespoon olive oil, plus 1 teaspoon**

**1 teaspoon red wine vinegar**

**¾ teaspoon chili powder**

**¾ teaspoon ground cumin**

**½ teaspoon kosher salt**

**¼ teaspoon garlic powder**

Preheat the oven to 375°F. Line a baking sheet with aluminum foil.

Rinse and drain the chickpeas and blot with a paper towel or dish towel to remove all the lingering moisture. Don't skip this step or your chickpeas won't get as crunchy.

In a small bowl, mix the 1 tablespoon oil, vinegar, chili powder, cumin, salt, and garlic powder.

Arrange the dried chickpeas on the baking sheet and pour the olive oil mixture over the top. Using your hands, mix together to make sure all the chickpeas are coated with the oil and spices. Spread out evenly, making sure the chickpeas do not touch one another. Bake until the chickpeas are just crispy and feel lighter but are not burned, about 25 minutes. Toss with the 1 teaspoon oil and continue to bake for 5 minutes more. Allow the chickpeas to cool completely before eating. Eat right away, or store for up to 1 day in a sealed container.

Per serving: 146 calories, 6 g protein, 19 g carbohydrates, 4 g fiber, <1 g total sugar, 5 g fat, <1 g saturated fat, 173 mg sodium, 20 mg potassium (1% DV), 53 mg calcium (5% DV), 2 mg magnesium (1% DV), 0 mcg B12 (0% DV), 0.01 mg B6 (1% DV), 0.6 mg iron (4% DV)

# Lemon-Glazed Mini Zucchini Muffins

These muffins are moist and sweet like the kind you might find at a local coffee shop, with about half the sugar and more fiber. The glaze adds a lemon zing that makes them even more special.

makes 12 servings (24 mini muffins) / prep time: 10 minutes / total time: 35 minutes

## Muffins

**Cooking spray**

**1 cup whole wheat flour**

**½ cup almond meal or almond flour**

**1 teaspoon ground cinnamon**

**½ teaspoon baking powder**

**¼ teaspoon baking soda**

**¼ teaspoon ground nutmeg**

**2 large eggs**

**½ cup sugar**

**¼ cup coconut oil**

**¼ cup unsweetened applesauce**

**1 teaspoon pure vanilla extract**

**1 cup grated unpeeled zucchini**

**⅓ cup finely chopped walnuts**

## Glaze

**1 scant tablespoon freshly squeezed lemon juice**

**¼ cup powdered sugar**

Preheat the oven to 350°F. Spray a mini muffin tin with cooking spray or brush lightly with vegetable oil.

Combine the whole wheat flour, almond meal, cinnamon, baking powder, baking soda, and nutmeg and stir to combine. In a separate bowl, whisk together the eggs, sugar, oil, applesauce, and vanilla. Gently stir in the zucchini.

Make a well in the center of the bowl of the dry ingredients and gradually mix in the wet ingredients until fully combined. Stir in the walnuts.

Pour the batter into a mini muffin tin, for a total of 24 mini muffins. Bake until a toothpick inserted into the center of a mini muffin comes out clean, about 25 minutes. Let the muffins cool, then remove from the muffin tin.

To make the glaze, stir the lemon juice into the powdered sugar until the sugar has dissolved, then drizzle the glaze over the top of the muffins.

Per 2 muffins: 180 calories, 4 g protein, 20 g carbohydrates, 2 g fiber, 12 g total sugar, 4.0 g fat, 4.4 g saturated fat, 505 mg sodium, 1604 mg potassium (46% DV), 122 mg calcium (12% DV), 90 mg magnesium (22% DV), 0.2 mcg B12 (4% DV), 1.0 mg B6 (52% DV), 0.8 mg iron (4% DV)

# CHAPTER SEVEN

# I'm Exhausted: Meals You Can Whip Up in 30 Minutes or Less

You need fast meals when your feet are swollen and the pressure in your legs is building up—we completely understand. And we'll let you in on a secret—you'll need these meals from now on, because once that baby comes, your leisurely kitchen time tends to take a dive. It's totally possible to carve out time, but it sure is nice to have fast meals that don't require a lot of fuss to use on the regular. The meals in this chapter give you just that. They don't take more than 30 minutes from start to finish, and most take even less. They are so simple that even someone who's not too familiar around the kitchen can whip them up quickly.

Throughout the recipes, we've also noted shortcuts that you can take to make them easier and/or save even more time. Finally, these recipes are forgiving in terms of swaps. So, if you don't have one ingredient, swap it for another food in the same food group—for instance, banana for blueberries, shrimp for chicken, and walnuts for pecans.

# Blueberry-Sunflower Seed Overnight Oats

Soaking oats in milk overnight softens them so they're ready to eat with no fuss in the morning, which is especially helpful if your growing belly has you moving a bit more slowly in the a.m.! If you're skeptical about eating uncooked oats, trust us on this one—when soaked overnight the texture of the oats is very similar to the cooked version.

---

makes 2 servings / prep time: 5 minutes / total time: 5 minutes + at least 6 hours of refrigeration

1 cup old-fashioned rolled oats

1⅓ cups 1% milk or unsweetened dairy-free alternative

1 teaspoon pure vanilla extract

1 teaspoon pure maple syrup or honey

Dash of coarse sea salt

2 cups blueberries (fresh or frozen and thawed)

2 tablespoons roasted unsalted sunflower seeds

Combine the oats, milk, vanilla, maple syrup, and salt in a bowl or jar with a lid (canning jars work really well and can serve as a to-go container, too). Cover and let sit in the refrigerator overnight. In the morning top each serving with the blueberries and sunflower seeds.

*Note:* You can heat this in the microwave if you prefer it as hot cereal, although we also love it cold, straight out of the fridge.

Per serving: 372 calories, 14 g protein, 61 g carbohydrates, 8 g fiber, 26 g total sugar, 9 g fat, 1.9 g saturated fat, 77 mg sodium, 571 mg potassium (16% DV), 112 mg magnesium (28% DV), 0.763 mcg B12 (13% DV), 0.296 mg B6 (15% DV), 2.6 mg iron (15% DV)

# Figs in a Blanket

Dried figs are tucked into almond butter and wrapped in a crisp but warm tortilla, making this easy 5-minute breakfast taste like something a bit more special, without the hassle.

makes 1 serving / prep time: 5 minutes / total time: 5 minutes

**1 teaspoon coconut oil**

**1½ tablespoons salted natural almond butter**

**1 (8-inch) whole grain tortilla**

**1 large dried fig (such as the Calimyrna variety), sliced**

**½ teaspoon brown sugar or maple syrup**

**Dash of ground cinnamon**

Heat the oil in a medium skillet over medium-high heat. Spread the almond butter evenly over one side of the tortilla. Distribute the fig slices over one half of the almond butter–spread tortilla. Sprinkle with the brown sugar and cinnamon and fold the tortilla in half. Place the folded tortilla in the skillet with the heated oil and cook on each side until browned, about 1½ minutes per side.

Per serving: 355 calories, 9 g protein, 41 g carbohydrates, 6 g fiber, 7 g total sugar, 20 g fat, 5.5 g saturated fat, 362 mg sodium, 367 mg potassium (10% DV), 94 mg calcium (9% DV), 119 mg magnesium (30% DV), 0 mcg B12 (0% DV), 0.117 mg B6 (9% DV), 2 mg iron (11% DV)

# 3-Minute Salsa and Cheddar Microwave Egg Sandwich

  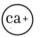 

This egg sandwich comes together in less time than it takes to wait in line at a fast-food restaurant, and provides nutrient-packed, protein-rich calories for your growing little one. Salsa adds flavor and some veggies to your breakfast, while the English muffin provides high-fiber carbs in the right portion size compared to most dine-out breakfast options.

makes 1 sandwich / prep time: 5 minutes / total time: 5 minutes

**1 teaspoon olive oil**

**1 large egg**

**1 teaspoon water**

**Dash of garlic powder**

**Dash of freshly ground black pepper**

**3 tablespoons shredded cheddar cheese**

**Whole wheat English muffin, halved and toasted**

**1 tablespoon salsa**

Spray or swirl the oil in a 3- to 4-inch diameter shallow bowl or ramekin. Crack the egg into the bowl and whisk with the water, garlic powder, and pepper. Microwave at full power for 45 seconds. Flip the egg over with a fork, then microwave for another 15 seconds. Add the cheese, and microwave for another 15 seconds. Remove the egg from the bowl, place on an English muffin, and top with the salsa.

Per serving: 335 calories, 18 g protein, 29 g carbohydrates, 5 g fiber, 6 g total sugar, 18 g fat, 7 g saturated fat, 570 mg sodium, 828 mg potassium (8% DV), 362 mg calcium (36% DV), 62 mg magnesium (16% DV), 0.621 mcg B12 (10% DV), 0.621 mg B6 (12% DV), 2.7 mg iron (15% DV)

# Black Bean Quesadillas

These quick quesadillas combine three satisfying textures in one single dish. They have all the makings of a nutritionally balanced and satisfying meal in 20 minutes, using common pantry staples. Better yet, give your feet a rest and hand off the recipe to your significant other. Even if they aren't too comfy in the kitchen, this recipe is simple enough to master on the first try! Serve with a side of steamed veggies or a green salad to round out the meal.

makes 4 servings (1 quesadilla per serving) / prep time: 10 minutes / total time: 20 minutes

---

**4 teaspoons olive oil, divided**

**1 green bell pepper, chopped**

**2 teaspoons minced garlic**

**1 (15-ounce) can black beans, rinsed and drained**

**1 cup frozen corn kernels, thawed**

**¼ cup salsa**

**½ teaspoon ground cumin**

**½ teaspoon sea salt, divided**

**¼ teaspoon garlic powder**

**¼ cup chopped fresh cilantro, plus more for garnish**

**1 avocado, sliced**

**1 teaspoon freshly squeezed lime juice**

**4 (10-inch) whole wheat tortillas**

**¼ cup 0% plain Greek yogurt**

Heat 2 teaspoons of the oil in a large skillet over medium-high heat. Add the bell pepper and sauté until softened, 3 to 4 minutes. Add the garlic and cook until fragrant, about 1 minute more. Add the beans, corn, salsa, cumin, ¼ teaspoon of the salt, garlic powder, stirring until well combined. Cook until the beans and corn are hot, stirring a couple of times, 5 minutes. Turn off the heat and, using a potato masher or fork, mash the bean mixture until about half of the beans are mashed. Stir in the cilantro. In a small bowl, mash the avocado with the lime juice and the remaining ¼ teaspoon salt.

Spread half of each tortilla with the bean and veggie mixture, then cover with avocado. Fold each tortilla in half, pressing gently to seal. Heat the remaining 2 teaspoons oil in the skillet. Cook each quesadilla until crispy, about 2 minutes per side. Top each with 1 tablespoon of yogurt and cilantro, if desired.

Per serving: 420 calories, 17 g protein, 68 g carbohydrates, 16 g fiber, 4 g total sugar, 11 g fat, 2 g saturated fat, 556 mg sodium, 542 mg potassium (15% DV), 52 mg calcium (5% DV), 85 mg magnesium (21% DV), 0 mcg B12 (0% DV), 0.337 mg B6 (17% DV), 10.4 mg iron (58% DV)

# Goat Cheese, Roasted Pepper, Spinach, and Herb Frittata

Frittatas are a great way to take eggs up a notch for dinner. In this recipe, rich goat cheese complements sweet roasted peppers and delicate baby spinach to make a hearty meal out of eggs. Serve it with whole grain toast points sprayed with olive oil and sprinkled with garlic powder, and a side salad for a balanced meal.

makes 2 servings / prep time: 10 minutes / total time: 20 minutes

**6 large whole eggs**

**4 large egg whites**

**2 tablespoons torn fresh basil leaves**

**2 tablespoons chopped fresh chives**

**1 tablespoon chopped fresh flat-leaf parsley**

**1 tablespoon water**

**½ teaspoon dried oregano**

**2 teaspoons olive oil**

**¾ cup chopped roasted peppers**

**⅔ cup crumbled goat cheese**

Preheat the oven to 350°F.

Whisk together the eggs, egg whites, basil, chives, parsley, water, and oregano in a medium bowl. Heat the oil in a 10- to 12-inch skillet over medium heat for 1 minute. Pour in the egg mixture and sprinkle the roasted peppers and goat cheese evenly over the top of the frittata. Cook until the bottom layer has set, 3 to 5 minutes. Transfer to the oven and cook until the eggs are cooked through, about 10 minutes. Cut the frittata into wedges and serve.

Per serving: 236 calories, 19 g protein, 3 g carbohydrates, 1 g fiber, 2 g total sugar, 17 g fat, 7 g saturated fat, 257 mg sodium, 231 mg potassium (7% DV), 147 mg calcium (15% DV), 24 mg magnesium (6% DV), 1.039 mcg B12 (17% DV), 0.22 mg B6 (11% DV), 3.1 mg iron (17% DV)

# Soba Noodles with Edamame and Sesame-Peanut Sauce

Take 20 minutes to make this recipe over the weekend, and you'll have four tasty, nutrient-packed lunches or dinners ready when you need 'em. This dish gets even better after it's been in the fridge overnight, and will satisfy that craving for takeout!

makes 4 servings / prep time: 10 minutes / total time: 20 minutes

## Salad

- **4 ounces soba (buckwheat) noodles or whole wheat spaghetti**
- **2 teaspoons extra-virgin olive oil**
- **2 cups frozen shelled edamame, thawed**
- **1 medium red bell pepper, diced**
- **1 cup grated or julienned carrots**
- **¼ cup sliced scallions**
- **2 tablespoons chopped fresh cilantro leaves**
- **2 tablespoons sesame seeds**

## Peanut Sauce

- **1 large garlic clove, minced**
- **2 tablespoons toasted sesame oil**
- **2 tablespoons creamy natural peanut butter**
- **2 tablespoons low-sodium soy sauce or tamari**
- **1 tablespoon rice vinegar**
- **2 teaspoons brown sugar**
- **2 teaspoons grated fresh ginger**
- **1 teaspoon sriracha sauce (optional)**
- **1 tablespoon warm water, or more as needed**

Cook the noodles according to the package directions. While the noodles are cooking, combine all the ingredients for the peanut sauce in a small bowl and whisk until smooth. Drain the noodles, saving some of the pasta cooking water to thin out the sauce, if desired.

Transfer the noodles to a large bowl, and toss with the oil, edamame, bell pepper, and carrots. Pour the peanut sauce over the ingredients in the bowl and toss until well combined. Top with the scallions, cilantro, and sesame seeds.

Per serving: 345 calories, 17 g protein, 40 g carbohydrates, 10 g fiber, 8 g total sugar, 15 g fat, 2.5 g saturated fat, 299 mg sodium, 659 mg potassium (19% DV), 90 mg calcium (9% DV), 130 mg magnesium (33% DV), 0 mcg B12 (0% DV), 0.343 mg B6 (17% DV), 4.2 mg iron (23% DV)

# Lemon-Herb Faux Egg Salad Pita Pocket

     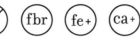

For the vegan moms-to-be, or anyone with some tofu in the fridge and/or a willingness to try new things, this faux egg salad tastes similar to traditional egg salad with a tangy flavor and a crunchy celery finish. It's the perfect complement to a toasted whole wheat pita with arugula (or any other salad green) for lunch. Serve with a piece of fruit to complete your meal.

makes 4 servings / prep time: 10 minutes / total time: 10 minutes

½ cup mayonnaise or vegan mayo

2 tablespoons Dijon mustard

1 teaspoon freshly squeezed lemon juice

¼ teaspoon ground turmeric

¼ teaspoon garlic powder

¼ teaspoon sea salt

¼ teaspoon cayenne pepper

1 (14-ounce) package firm tofu, drained well and diced into small cubes or mashed

½ cup chopped celery

¼ cup scallions

2 tablespoons chopped fresh flat-leaf parsley, or 1 teaspoon dried

1 tablespoon chopped fresh dill

4 (6-inch) whole wheat pitas

1 cup arugula

In a small bowl, whisk together the mayonnaise, mustard, lemon juice, turmeric, garlic powder, salt, and cayenne.

Combine the tofu, celery, scallions, parsley, and dill in a medium bowl, add the mayonnaise mixture, and toss to coat. Chill the salad for 1 to 2 hours. Serve stuffed into pita with the arugula.

Per serving (1 sandwich) : 460 calories, 16 g protein, 40 g carbohydrates, 6 g fiber, 2 g total sugar, 28 g fat, 4 g saturated fat, 636 mg sodium, 212 mg potassium (6% DV), 215 mg calcium (22% DV), 55 mg magnesium (14% DV), 0.091 mcg B12 (2% DV), 0.361 mg B6 (18% DV), 3.8 mg iron (21% DV)

# Turkey Ragu–Topped Baked Potatoes

   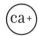

This is an Italian spin on a chili-topped baked potato. Try it to give your weeknight rotation a little variation!

makes 4 servings / prep time: 5 minutes / total time: 30 minutes

1 tablespoon olive oil, plus 1 teaspoon

1 cup chopped onion

1 cup grated carrots (save time by using pre-grated bagged carrots)

2 garlic cloves, minced

1 pound lean ground turkey breast

2 tablespoons tomato paste

1 (28-ounce) can crushed tomatoes (such as San Marzano)

2 teaspoons dried oregano

½ teaspoon salt

½ teaspoon freshly ground black pepper

¼ teaspoon red pepper flakes (optional)

4 medium baking potatoes (russet)

½ cup grated Parmesan cheese

¼ cup chopped fresh flat-leaf parsley

Heat the 1 tablespoon oil in a medium skillet over medium-high heat, add the onion and carrots and cook until soft and lightly browned, about 10 minutes. Add the garlic and cook until fragrant and golden, 1 minute more. Remove the mixture from the skillet and set aside.

In the same skillet, heat the 1 teaspoon oil, add the turkey and cook over medium heat, break apart with a spoon, until browned, about 6 minutes.

Stir in the tomato paste and cook 2 minutes more. Add the tomatoes, oregano, salt, black pepper, and red pepper flakes (if using). Return the onion and carrot mixture to the skillet and bring to a boil. Reduce the heat and simmer until most of the liquid has cooked down, about 10 minutes.

While the sauce cooks, poke multiple holes in the potatoes using a fork. Microwave each potato until the flesh is fork-tender, about 4 minutes. Cut the potatoes lengthwise down the middle and mash the flesh gently with a fork, without tearing the skin, to provide nooks and crannies to absorb the sauce. Top each potato with the turkey sauce. Top with the Parmesan and parsley.

Per serving: 492 calories, 34 g protein, 53 g carbohydrates, 11 g fiber, 12 g total sugar, 17 g fat, 5 g saturated fat, 650 mg sodium, 1607 mg potassium (46% DV), 224 mg calcium (22% DV), 86 mg magnesium (22% DV), 1.642 mcg B12 (27% DV), 0.956 mg B6 (48% DV), 5 mg iron (28% DV)

# Spanish-Style Garlic Shrimp

Shrimp is an excellent source of protein. Keep a bag of shrimp in your freezer to have a lean, delicious protein that cooks in less than 10 minutes. They're easy and fast to defrost. Buying frozen is actually just as good as "fresh." Unless you live in an area with fresh shrimp, even the "fresh" shrimp at the fish market has typically already been frozen and thawed. Serve over brown rice or quinoa, with a side of steamed veggies or a salad, or over mixed greens with a light vinaigrette.

makes 2 servings / prep time: 10 minutes / total time: 20 minutes

**4 garlic cloves, divided**

**½ pound large shrimp, peeled and deveined**

**4½ teaspoons olive oil, divided**

**¼ teaspoon sweet paprika**

**¼ teaspoon red pepper flakes**

**2 teaspoons red wine vinegar**

**¼ teaspoon salt**

**2 tablespoons coarsely chopped fresh flat-leaf parsley**

Mince 2 of the garlic cloves. In a medium bowl or a zip-top bag, toss the shrimp with the minced garlic, 2 teaspoons of the oil, and the paprika. Let sit while you continue the other steps.

Add the remaining 2½ teaspoons oil to a medium skillet over medium-high heat. Smash the remaining 2 garlic cloves with the flat side of a knife (the cloves should be mostly flattened), then add to the oil, along with the red pepper flakes. Cook the garlic until browned, but not burned, swirling the oil around a couple of times to coat the garlic, 2 to 3 minutes. Remove the garlic with a fork or slotted spoon, leaving the oil behind.

Add the shrimp to the pan of oil, spacing them out evenly. Cook on one side until the shrimp begins to turn opaque, about 1 minute. Flip the shrimp and cook until the second side is cooked, about another minute. Add the vinegar and salt, stirring to remove the brown bits from the pan, and reduce the heat to medium. Cook for another minute, then toss with the parsley to coat. Serve immediately.

Per serving: 197 calories, 23 g protein, 2 g carbohydrates, 0 g fiber, 0 g total sugar, 11 g fat, 1.5 g saturated fat, 179 mg sodium, 345 mg potassium (10% DV), 89 mg calcium (9% DV), 43 mg magnesium (11% DV), 0 mcg B12 (0% DV), 0.77 mg B6 (39% DV), 0.3 mg iron (2% DV)

Healthy, Happy Pregnancy Cookbook

# Penne with Greens and Chicken Sausage

This easy, 30-minute pasta dish features flavorful Italian chicken sausage and Swiss chard, which come together with tangy sun-dried tomatoes and a generous sprinkling of Parmesan cheese.

makes 4 servings / prep time: 10 minutes / total time: 30 minutes

**4 teaspoons olive oil, divided**

**4 pre-cooked Italian chicken sausages, cut into ½-inch slices**

**1 bunch Swiss chard, stems and leaves separated and chopped**

**1 (14-ounce) can artichoke hearts in water, drained**

**3 garlic cloves, minced**

**¼ teaspoon freshly ground black pepper**

**⅓ cup thinly sliced sun-dried tomatoes (not oil-packed)**

**3 cups dry whole wheat penne**

**1 tablespoon tomato paste**

**⅓ cup chopped fresh basil leaves**

**¼ teaspoon red pepper flakes**

**¾ cup grated Parmesan cheese**

Bring a large pot of water to a boil for the pasta. Meanwhile, heat 2 teaspoons of the oil in a large skillet over medium heat. Add the sausage and cook until just browned on each side, about 3 minutes. Remove from the skillet and set aside.

To the same skillet, add the remaining 2 teaspoons oil, the chard stems, artichoke hearts, garlic, and black pepper. Cook until the chard stems soften slightly, 3 to 5 minutes.

Add the chard leaves and cook, stirring, until wilted, 3 to 5 minutes more. Stir the sun-dried tomatoes into to the chard mixture and remove from the heat.

Cook the pasta until al dente according to the package directions. Reserve 1 cup of the pasta cooking water, drain the pasta, and return it to the pot.

Whisk the tomato paste and reserved pasta water in a small bowl. Reduce the heat to low and add the tomato paste mixture and sausage to the chard mixture in the skillet. Stir to combine. Remove from the heat. Stir in the basil, red pepper flakes, and pasta and top with Parmesan.

Per serving: 545 calories, 34 g protein, 75 g carbohydrates, 13 g fiber, 5 g total sugar, 16 g fat, 5 g saturated fat, 850 mg sodium, 777 mg potassium (18% DV), 294 mg calcium (29% DV), 201 mg magnesium (50% DV), 0.424 mcg B12 (7% DV), 0.341 mg B6 (17% DV), 2.2 mg iron (12% DV)

# 10-Minute Maple-Mustard Salmon

Eating fish is so important for health, especially omega-3-rich fatty fish like salmon. But many people shy away from eating it regularly because they're unsure how to prepare it. This recipe is simple as can be, only takes 10 minutes from start to finish, and is loaded with omega-3 fats. Serve with a whole grain like brown rice or quinoa and a side of roasted or steamed vegetables.

makes 2 servings / prep time: 5 minutes / total time: 10 minutes

1 tablespoon Dijon or grainy mustard

2 teaspoons maple syrup

1 teaspoon freshly squeezed lemon juice

1 teaspoon chopped fresh rosemary, or ¼ teaspoon dried

8 ounces salmon fillet, skin on or off

¼ teaspoon kosher salt

¼ teaspoon freshly ground black pepper

1 tablespoon chopped, fresh flat-leaf parsley (optional)

Preheat the broiler to high.

Whisk the mustard, maple syrup, lemon juice, and rosemary together in a small bowl.

Place the fillet on a baking sheet lined with foil. Sprinkle the top of the fish with the salt and pepper. Brush the mustard mix over the top and sides of the fillet. Broil on high, skin side down if the fish has skin, until the salmon is just cooked through, about 8 minutes. Sprinkle with parsley, if using.

Per serving: 196 calories, 23 g protein, 6 g carbohydrates, 0.5 g fiber, 5 g total sugar, 8 g fat, 1 g saturated fat, 192 mg sodium, 609 mg potassium (13% DV), 32 mg calcium (3% DV), 48 mg magnesium (12% DV), 3.6 mcg B12 (150% DV), 0.9 mg B6 (73% DV), 1.3 mg iron (8% DV)

# Shrimp Tacos with Mango-Spinach Salsa

Using bold flavors like Cajun seasonings, lime, cilantro, and mango allows this dish to have simple ingredients and a fast prep to table time with BIG flavor. What's even better than how delicious it is, is how easy it is. So even if baby is fussy, at least your dinner isn't! Don't be intimidated if the ingredient list looks long, it's mostly spices and there's a shortcut for that, too. Serve with a side salad or a side of steamed veggies for a complete meal.

makes 4 servings (2 tacos per serving) / prep time: 10 minutes / total time: 20 minutes

1¼ pounds frozen uncooked shrimp, thawed, peeled, and deveined

1 teaspoon ground cumin (see Note)

½ teaspoon garlic powder

½ teaspoon sea salt, divided

½ teaspoon freshly ground black pepper, divided

¼ teaspoon cayenne pepper

1 mango, peeled and cut into cubes

1 cup grape tomatoes, halved

1 cup chopped baby spinach

2 teaspoons minced garlic, divided

¼ cup chopped fresh cilantro, divided

Juice of 2 limes, divided

1 tablespoon olive oil

½ cup 2% plain Greek yogurt

8 (6-inch) corn tortillas

1 avocado, cut into cubes

Pat the shrimp dry and toss with the cumin, garlic powder, ¼ teaspoon of the salt, ¼ teaspoon of the black pepper, and the cayenne until thoroughly coated. Set aside while you make the salsa.

In a medium bowl, combine the mango, grape tomatoes, spinach, 1 teaspoon of the garlic, 2 tablespoons of the cilantro, the juice of 1 lime, and the remaining ¼ teaspoon each salt and black pepper.

Heat the oil in a medium skillet over medium-high heat. Add the shrimp and cook until the shrimp begins to turn opaque, about 1 minute. Flip to the other side and add the remaining teaspoon garlic, tossing to coat. Cook until just pink, another minute. Remove the shrimp from the heat and toss with juice of the remaining 1 lime.

Place a drizzle of the yogurt along the length of each tortilla, add the shrimp, then top with salsa, avocado, and the remaining cilantro.

*Note:* Short (er) cut. If you don't have time to mix up the spices (it only takes about 1 minute, but we get it!), substitute 1 tablespoon Cajun seasoning instead of the cumin through black pepper.

Per serving: 400 calories, 27 g protein, 45 g carbohydrates, 8.5 g fiber, 16 g total sugar, 15 g fat, 3 g saturated fat, 603 mg sodium, 796 mg potassium (17% DV), 204 mg calcium (20% DV), 101 mg magnesium (25% DV), 1.5 mcg B12 (66% DV), 0.6 mg B6 (49% DV), 1.6 mg iron (9% DV)

# Cucumber-Sesame Salad

This cool, refreshing side salad can be made ahead (it's even better the next day!) and acts as a quick, no-cook vegetable side. Comprised of 95 percent water, cucumbers are also a great source of hydration to help meet your increasing water needs.

makes 2 servings / prep time: 10 minutes / total time: 10 minutes

1 tablespoon rice vinegar

1 teaspoon toasted sesame oil

1 teaspoon olive oil

1 teaspoon honey

⅛ teaspoon garlic powder

⅛ teaspoon salt

2 cups thinly sliced cucumbers

¼ cup very thinly sliced red onion

1 tablespoon sesame seeds

In a medium bowl, whisk together the vinegar, sesame oil, olive oil, honey, garlic powder, and salt. Add the cucumbers and onion and toss to coat. Sprinkle with the sesame seeds. Chill before serving or eat immediately.

Per serving: 100 calories, 2 g protein, 8 g carbohydrates, 2 g fiber, 5 g total sugar, 7 g fat, 1 g saturated fat, 76 mg sodium, 214 mg potassium (5% DV), 27 mg calcium (3%,DV), 32 mg magnesium (8% DV), 0 mcg B12 (0% DV), .09 mg B6 (7% DV), 0.3 mg iron (1% DV)

# Microwave Apple Crisp with Walnuts

An apple crisp might not immediately pop into your mind when you think of fast food, but it will now! This crisp is made in the microwave in less than 10 minutes. So, you can crave homemade apple crisp and be noshing soft cinnamony apples topped with buttery, nutty oat crumble just minutes later.

makes 2 servings / prep time: 5 minutes / total time: 10 minutes

1 tablespoon unsalted butter, plus 2 teaspoons

2 tablespoons old-fashioned rolled oats

3 teaspoons brown sugar, divided

3 teaspoons whole wheat flour, divided

1 tablespoon chopped walnuts

1 large apple, sliced

¼ teaspoon ground cinnamon

Cooking spray or oil

2 tablespoons vanilla ice cream

In a small microwave-safe bowl, microwave the 1 tablespoon butter until melted, about 45 seconds. Stir in the oats, 2 teaspoons of the sugar, 2 teaspoons of the flour, and the walnuts, until the topping resembles crumbs. Set aside.

Toss the apple slices with the cinnamon, the remaining 1 teaspoon sugar, and the remaining 1 teaspoon flour. Spray two ramekins, 3 or 4 inches in diameter, with cooking spray or rub with oil. Lay half the apple slices on the bottom of each ramekin and top each with the 1 teaspoon butter, then top with the oat crumble. Microwave each crisp until the apples are soft, about 1½ minutes. Top each with 1 tablespoon of ice cream.

Per serving: 206 calories, 4 g protein, 24 g carbohydrates, 3 g fiber, 15 g total sugar, 13 g fat, 6.5 g saturated fat, 13 mg sodium, 153 mg potassium (4% DV), 47 mg calcium (5% DV), 23 mg magnesium (6% DV), 0.01 mcg B12 (0% DV), .09 mg B6 (5% DV), 0.6 mg iron (3% DV)

# Dark Chocolate Mug Brownie

What's better than a brownie? One you can make in less than 5 minutes whenever the craving strikes! This fudgy dessert is what we'd imagine the baby of brownie batter and a cooked brownie would be. Try one when your next chocolate craving hits. Bonus: since you won't be baking a whole batch, there's no temptation to keep eating out of the pan!

makes 1 brownie / prep time: 5 minutes / total time: 5 minutes

Cooking spray or oil

2 tablespoons whole wheat flour (or substitute almond flour for a gluten-free version)

2 tablespoons unsweetened cocoa powder

2 teaspoons brown sugar

2 teaspoons dark chocolate chips

Dash of ground cinnamon

2 tablespoons unsweetened almond milk

2 teaspoons coconut oil, melted

Splash of pure vanilla extract

Spray a 12-ounce coffee mug with cooking spray or rub lightly with oil. In the prepared mug, stir in the flour, cocoa powder, sugar, chocolate chips, and cinnamon until evenly dispersed. Add the almond milk, coconut oil, and vanilla and stir to create a batter. Be careful not to overmix or the brownie will be rubbery. Microwave 1 to 1½ minutes until the cake is just firm—it will be gooier than a traditional brownie.

Turn the brownie out of the mug onto a plate to serve, or spoon it right out of the mug and nosh away.

Per serving: 220 calories, 5 g protein, 27 g carbohydrates, 6 g fiber, 10 g total sugar, 13 g fat, 10 g saturated fat, 35 mg sodium, 255 mg potassium, 111 mg calcium (11%,DV), 86 mg magnesium (22% DV), 0.562 mcg B12 (9% DV), .079 mg B6 (4% DV), 2.3 mg iron (13% DV)

# Paper Bag Microwave Popcorn

This technique takes 3 minutes (the same amount of time it would take to make a bag of store-bought microwave popcorn), it's free of additives, and gives you a blank canvas on which to create your topping and flavor combinations.

makes 1 serving / prep time: 1 minute / total time: 4 minutes

**3 tablespoons popcorn kernels**

**1 teaspoon olive oil**

**Brown paper lunch bag**

**Dash of kosher salt**

**Dash of freshly ground black pepper**

Toss the kernels in the oil and place in a brown paper lunch bag. Fold the top of the bag over about 1/2 inch, two to three times to make sure it stays closed. Microwave on high until the popcorn popping slows to 3 seconds between each pop, 2 to 2½ minutes. Add salt and pepper to the bag and shake to combine.

Per serving: 160 calories, 4 g protein, 29 g carbohydrates, 6 g fiber, 0 g total sugar, 6 g fat, 0.5 g saturated fat, 68 mg sodium, 1 mg potassium (0% DV), 0.5 mg calcium (0%,DV), 0 mg magnesium (0% DV), 0 mcg B12 (0% DV), 0 mg B6 (0% DV), 1.1 mg iron (6% DV)

# Finding the Healthiest Frozen Meals

There are some great frozen meal options out there, but there are also some real duds. Use these criteria to make sure that when you do opt for frozen meals, you're getting the best there is.

**Frozen Breakfast Sandwich or Wrap (per item)**

- At least 3 g fiber
- No more than 5 g saturated fat
- At least 10 g protein
- No more than 500 mg sodium
- No partially hydrogenated oils

**Frozen Burrito (per burrito)**

- 2 g saturated fat or less
- At least 4 g fiber
- At least 8 g protein
- 500 mg or less sodium
- No partially hydrogenated oils/trans fat

**Frozen Pizza (per serving)**

- No more than 4.5 g saturated fat
- No more than 700 mg sodium
- At least 4 g fiber
- No partially hydrogenated oils/trans fats

**Gluten-Free Frozen Pizza (per serving)**

- No more than 5 g saturated fat
- No more than 700 mg sodium
- At least 2 g fiber
- No partially hydrogenated oils/trans fats

# I Won't Have This Much Free Time for a Very Long Time: Prep Ahead Recipes Before Baby

In the first weeks (okay who are we kidding, months) after baby comes, cooking will most likely be the last thing you want to, or have time to, do. The goal of these recipes is to stock your freezer with meals and snacks that still taste great after being frozen and reheated, will satisfy your hunger and new nutrition needs, and that you can easily thaw and eat (with one hand if you need to). There's a mix of your typical freezer fare, such as casserole-style dishes and soups, as well as patties, burgers, and even egg muffins. We squeezed lots of veggies into most of these dishes so that just in case you can't heat some up in the micro, you're not lacking.

Don't stress about making everything, and certainly do enlist the help of friends and family who offer. If they don't already have something in mind, now you have recipes to recommend!

In addition to being freezer friendly, these meals are all nutritionally balanced and offer a combination of protein, healthy fats, and fiber to help keep your energy up when you need it most.

# Berry, Banana, and Greens Smoothie Bag

You'll appreciate the convenience factor in both making and drinking this breakfast once baby arrives. This smoothie packs in everything you need for a healthy breakfast, including protein, calcium, and even a serving of veggies. But with the prep work done, all you have to do is empty the bag of ingredients into the blender, add milk and yogurt, and blend. You've got this in the bag . . . (we couldn't resist!).

---

makes 2 servings / prep time: 5 minutes / total time: 8 minutes

**2 cups baby spinach or kale**

**1 cup frozen strawberries**

**1 banana, peeled and cut into chunks**

**1 tablespoon unsweetened shredded coconut**

**1 cup 1% milk, skim milk, or unsweetened dairy-free alternative**

**⅔ cup low-fat plain yogurt or unsweetened dairy-free alternative**

Add the spinach, strawberries, banana chunks, and coconut to a 1-quart freezer bag and store in the freezer. When ready to sip, add the milk to a blender, then the smoothie bag contents, then the yogurt. Blend until smooth.

*Note:* If you don't have a powerful blender, we recommend blending the greens with the milk first, until thoroughly combined. Then add the rest of the smoothie bag ingredients and the yogurt and blend until smooth.

Per serving: 394 calories, 19 g protein, 68 g carbohydrates, 9 g fiber, 44 g total sugar, 8 g fat, 6 g saturated fat, 247 mg sodium, 1676 mg potassium (36% DV), 629 mg calcium (63% DV), 146 mg magnesium (37% DV), 1.8 mcg B12 (76% DV), 0.7 mg B6 (7% DV), 3.8 mg iron (21% DV)

# Whole Wheat Banana Nut Bread

    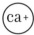

This bread has all of the moist texture and comforting flavor of your favorite sweet bread, but packs in more fiber and nutrition, and much less sugar, than a traditional recipe, or one you would get at a coffee shop. Freeze it in individual slices that you can thaw in the microwave and eat with one hand while holding baby. Nosh as a breakfast, pair with a latte, and you've got a complete meal.

makes 8 servings / prep time: 15 minutes / total time: 1 hour

2 large very ripe bananas, or 3 small, mashed (about 1 cup)

2 large eggs

½ cup packed brown sugar

¼ cup oil (grapeseed, safflower, olive, melted coconut, and sunflower seed all work well)

½ cup low-fat buttermilk (or ½ cup low-fat milk or unsweetened dairy-free alternative mixed with 2¼ teaspoons freshly squeezed lemon juice or vinegar)

1 teaspoon pure vanilla extract

1¼ cups whole wheat pastry flour

½ cup almond meal or finely ground almonds

½ teaspoon baking soda

1¼ teaspoons baking powder

¾ teaspoon ground cinnamon

½ teaspoon sea salt

¼ teaspoon ground nutmeg

⅓ cup chopped walnuts

Preheat the oven to 350°F. Lightly grease a 9 x 5-inch loaf pan.

In a large bowl, add the mashed bananas, and then whisk in the eggs, sugar, oil, buttermilk, and vanilla.

In a medium bowl, whisk together the flour, almond meal, baking soda, baking powder, cinnamon, salt, and nutmeg to combine. Fold half of the dry ingredients into the wet ingredients. Add the walnuts to the remaining dry ingredients, then add the dry ingredients to the wet ingredients until just combined.

Pour the batter into the loaf pan. Bake until the top is browned and a toothpick inserted into the center comes out clean, about 1 hour.

Per serving: 307 calories, 7 g protein, 38 g carbohydrates, 4 g fiber, 19 g total sugar, 15 g fat, 1.5 g saturated fat, 239 mg sodium, 272 mg potassium (6% DV), 117 mg calcium (11% DV), 68 mg magnesium (17% DV), 0.145 mcg B12 (6% DV), .26 mg B6 (20% DV), 1.6 mg iron (9% DV)

# Strawberry-Chia Pudding Breakfast Pops

These bars are the makings of the popular chia pudding, in a frozen pop format! Pull one out of the freezer whenever you are craving something cool, sweet, and interesting!

makes 6 pops / prep time: 10 minutes / total time: 10 minutes + overnight

2 cups low-fat plain kefir

2 cups fresh or frozen strawberries, slightly thawed (they'll be easier to blend)

2 tablespoons honey

½ teaspoon pure vanilla extract

⅓ cup chia seeds

Blend the kefir, strawberries, and honey in a blender until smooth, about 1 minute. Pour into a bowl and whisk in the vanilla and chia seeds until well combined. Cover and refrigerate for at least 2 hours, and up to 8 hours.

Pour the chilled mixture into freezer pop molds and freeze overnight.

Remove the pops from the molds and store in a sealed bag for up to 1 month. Eat as a frozen pop, or defrost in a bowl in the refrigerator overnight and enjoy as cold pudding in the morning.

Per serving: 145 calories, 6 g protein, 20 g carbohydrates, 5 g fiber, 13 g total sugar, 5 g fat, 1 g saturated fat, 56 mg sodium, 305 mg potassium (9% DV), 226 mg calcium (23% DV), 61 mg magnesium (15% DV), 0.424 mcg B12 (7% DV), 0.148 mg B6 (7% DV), 0.3 mg iron (1.6% DV)

# Cheddar-Quinoa Egg Muffins

These breakfast muffins are like mini crustless quiches and contain all of the nutrition you need for a complete breakfast, thanks to quinoa, eggs, and veggies. They're portable and easy to grab all while holding baby or rushing out the door. Pull one out of the freezer, microwave, and enjoy within 60 seconds. Eat 2 to 3 muffins paired with a piece of fruit for breakfast or 1 to 2 for a snack.

makes 4 to 6 servings (12 muffins) / prep time: 15 minutes / total time: 45 minutes

Cooking spray or oil

6 large eggs

4 large egg whites, or ¾ cup

1 cup cooked quinoa

1 cup finely chopped broccoli (fresh or frozen and thawed)

¾ cup shredded cheddar cheese

2 tablespoons sliced scallions

1 tablespoon chopped fresh flat-leaf parsley

1 teaspoon olive oil

½ teaspoon garlic powder

½ teaspoon salt

¼ to ½ teaspoon freshly ground black pepper

Preheat the oven to 350°F. Line a standard 12-cup muffin tin with muffin wrappers sprayed with cooking spray, or directly spray the tins, or rub the tins lightly with oil.

Whisk together the eggs and egg whites. Add the remaining ingredients, quinoa through black pepper, and stir to combine thoroughly. Bake until the eggs are cooked through and a toothpick inserted into a muffin comes out clean, about 20 minutes. Let the muffins cool in the tin for 10 minutes.

Using a knife to loosen the edges, remove the muffins from the tin and continue to cool in the refrigerator for 30 minutes. Once cool, freeze the muffins in a large freezer bag for up to 3 months, or keep in the fridge for up to 3 days.

Per serving: 200 calories, 16 g protein, 9 g carbohydrates, 2 g fiber, 1 g total sugar, 11 g fat, 5 g saturated fat, 309 mg sodium, 243 mg potassium (7% DV), 150 mg calcium (15% DV), 38 mg magnesium (10% DV), 0.59 mcg B12 (25% DV), 0.18 mg B6 (14% DV), 2.2 mg iron (12% DV)

# Peanut Butter-Cocoa-Chocolate Chip Energy Bites

These no-bake bites are packed with healthy fats and fiber, the perfect combination to get you through a busy morning of diaper changing. And who can resist the chocolate and peanut butter pairing? Freeze them in a sealed bag and eat right out of the freezer, or let thaw to soften up a bit. Either way, they're simple to pop in your mouth and eat with one hand.

makes 8 servings (16 bites) / prep time: 5 minutes / total time: 10 minutes

¾ cup salted natural peanut butter

3 tablespoons unsweetened cocoa powder

1½ tablespoons honey

1 teaspoon pure vanilla extract

1 cup old-fashioned rolled oats

½ cup unsweetened shredded coconut

¼ cup mini chocolate chips

Mix the peanut butter, cocoa powder, honey, and vanilla together in a large bowl. Add the oats, coconut, and chocolate chips and stir until uniform.

Form the mixture into 16 balls, about 1 inch in diameter, and place on a wax paper–lined baking sheet or a plate. Refrigerate for 20 minutes, then freeze in a resealable freezer bag or container. These bites will stay fresh in the freezer for up to 3 months.

Per serving: 254 calories, 8 g protein, 21 g carbohydrates, 4 g fiber, 9 g total sugar, 18 g fat, 6 g saturated fat, 8 mg sodium, 272 mg potassium (8% DV), 21 mg calcium (2% DV), 72 mg magnesium (18% DV), 0 mcg B12 (0% DV), 0.161 mg B6 (8% DV), 2.2 mg iron (12% DV)

# Kale and Chicken Sausage Soup

This soup is hearty and nutritionally balanced enough to be a meal on its own. So, once it's thawed, you have dinner on the table in no time. Pair it with a simple green salad to round out the meal.

makes 6 servings / prep time: 10 minutes / total time: 20 minutes

1½ tablespoons extra-virgin olive oil

1 pound pre-cooked chicken sausage (such as Applegate Farms)

1½ cups chopped yellow onion

6 garlic cloves, minced

6 cups water

3 cups low-sodium chicken broth or homemade chicken stock

1 teaspoon kosher salt

3 pounds Yukon Gold potatoes, cut into ½-inch pieces

6 cups kale, stems removed, leaves coarsely chopped

1½ tablespoons apple cider vinegar

¼ teaspoon red pepper flakes (optional)

¼ teaspoon freshly ground black pepper

Heat the oil in a soup pot or Dutch oven over medium heat. Add the sausage and cook, rotating, until the skin is browned all over, about 7 minutes. Remove from the pot and set aside. Once the sausage is cool enough to handle, cut into slices.

Add the onion to the same pot and cook until translucent, about 5 minutes. Add the garlic and cook until fragrant, about 1 minute. Add the water, broth, and salt and bring to a boil. Add the potatoes, kale, sausage, vinegar, and red pepper flakes and reduce to a simmer, cover, and cook over medium-low heat until the potatoes are fork-tender, about 9 minutes more. (If you plan to freeze the soup, undercook the potatoes slightly; see Note.) Season with the black pepper.

*Note:* Freezing soup: Remove the pot from the heat and let the soup cool slightly, about 30 minutes. Portion the soup into containers based on the number of servings you plan to thaw at once. Leave at least an inch of room at the top of the container for the liquid to expand. Write the date on the container and store for up to 3 months.

Per serving: 368 calories, 24 g protein, 51 g carbohydrates, 6 g fiber, 7 g total sugar, 10 g fat, 2 g saturated fat, 751 mg sodium, 1535 mg potassium (44% DV), 143 mg calcium (14% DV), 87 mg magnesium (22% DV), 0.12 mcg B12 (2% DV), 0.664 mg B6 (33% DV), 4 mg iron (20% DV)

# Smoky Black Bean and Sweet Potato Burgers

These veggie burgers are sweet and smoky, and we think they may be even better after they're frozen. They're packed with high-fiber beans and antioxidant-rich sweet potatoes and great over a green salad for an easy lunch or dinner.

makes 6 servings / prep time: 15 minutes / total time: 1 hour

**2½ cups peeled and chopped sweet potatoes (about 2 large)**

**3 teaspoons olive oil, divided**

**1 teaspoon chili powder, divided**

**1 teaspoon smoked or sweet paprika, divided**

**½ teaspoon ground cumin, divided**

**½ teaspoon kosher salt, divided**

**½ teaspoon freshly ground black pepper, divided**

**1 cup cooked millet or quinoa**

**¼ cup chopped fresh cilantro**

**½ cup chopped red onion**

**1 (15-ounce) can black beans, rinsed and drained**

**1 cup frozen corn kernals, thawed and drained**

Preheat the oven to 400°F. Line a baking sheet with parchment paper or aluminum foil.

Toss the sweet potatoes with 2 teaspoons of the oil, ½ teaspoon of the chili powder, ½ teaspoon of the paprika, ¼ teaspoon of the cumin, ¼ teaspoon of the salt, and ¼ teaspoon of the pepper. Spread the sweet potatoes out evenly on the baking sheet. Bake until golden and soft, about 20 minutes.

Combine the roasted sweet potatoes with the remaining ½ teaspoon chili powder, ½ teaspoon paprika, ¼ teaspoon cumin, ¼ teaspoon salt, and ¼ teaspoon pepper, the millet, cilantro, onion, beans, and corn in a food processor and pulse until the mixture is partially mashed but still contains some chunks of beans and veggies.

Form the mixture into six 4-inch patties. Brush the patties with the remaining 1 teaspoon oil. Bake on the baking sheet, turning halfway through the baking time, until browned on each side, about 25 minutes.

Per serving: 188 calories, 7 g protein, 35 g carbohydrates, 8 g fiber, 4 g total sugar, 3 g fat, 0.5 g saturated fat, 178 mg sodium, 297 mg potassium (9% DV), 24 mg calcium (2% DV), 38 mg magnesium (10% DV), 0 mcg B12 (0% DV), 0.178 mg B6 (3% DV), 4.1 mg iron (22% DV)

# Chicken Black Bean Burritos

Frozen burritos are convenient and delicious, but many store-bought brands are high in sodium and not filled with the cleanest ingredients. This homemade version tastes a lot like the ones from the store, is made with quality ingredients, heats up in 2½ minutes, and can be eaten with one hand if need be!

makes 8 servings (8 burritos) / prep time: 10 minutes / total time: 45 minutes

**16 ounces boneless, skinless chicken breast, or 2 cups chopped or shredded cooked chicken**

**3 cups low-sodium chicken broth**

**1 celery stalk with leaves, cut in half or quarters**

**1 teaspoon olive oil**

**¾ cup chopped onion**

**1 large carrot, finely chopped**

**2 garlic cloves, minced**

**½ cup salsa**

**1 (15-ounce) can black beans, rinsed and drained**

**1 (15-ounce) can diced tomatoes, drained**

**½ teaspoon sea salt**

**¼ teaspoon freshly ground black pepper**

**¼ teaspoon ground cumin**

**¼ teaspoon garlic powder**

**½ cup coarsely chopped fresh cilantro, or 1 tablespoon dried**

**8 (10-inch) whole wheat tortillas**

**8 ounces grated cheddar cheese (about 2 cups)**

Add the chicken, broth, and celery to a medium pot; the broth should cover the chicken by at least 1 inch. Bring the broth to a boil, then reduce the heat and simmer until the chicken is cooked to an internal temperature of 165°F, about 15 minutes. Let cool, then cut into small chunks, or shred. If you're using pre-cooked chicken, skip this step.

Heat the oil in a large skillet over medium-high heat. Add the onion and carrot and sauté until soft, about 7 minutes. Add the garlic and cook until fragrant, about 2 minutes more. Stir in the salsa, beans, tomatoes, salt, pepper, cumin, garlic powder, and chicken. Let simmer to heat through and blend the flavors, about 5 minutes. Turn off the heat and stir in the cilantro.

Spoon an even amount of the filling into the center of each tortilla. Top with the cheese, then roll, tucking the ends in, burrito-style.

Wrap each burrito individually in plastic wrap and then place in a zip-top freezer bag for storage. To reheat, remove the plastic wrap and microwave on high for 2 to 2½ minutes, or until the inside is hot, turning once.

Per serving: 430 calories, 29 g protein, 50 g carbohydrates, 10 g fiber, 3 g total sugar, 12 g fat, 6.5 g saturated fat, 734 mg sodium, 564 mg potassium (12% DV), 231 mg calcium (23% DV), 76 mg magnesium (19% DV), 0.36 mcg B12 (15% DV), 0.6 mg B6 (46% DV), 7 mg iron (26% DV)

# Turkey Lentil Loaf

This version of meat loaf is graced with tender lentils, veggies, and fresh herbs, giving it a great flavor and packing it with lean protein and fiber. Serve sliced with a side of steamed green beans and the Cauliflower-Potato Mash with Mushroom Gravy (page 133) for a completely balanced meal.

makes 6 servings / prep time: 20 minutes / total time: 1 hour 20 minutes

½ tablespoon olive oil

1 medium onion, finely chopped

1 cup grated carrots

3 garlic cloves, minced

1 cup cooked brown or green lentils

¼ cup ketchup

2 teaspoons Worcestershire sauce

¾ teaspoon kosher salt

¼ teaspoon freshly ground black pepper

¾ cup whole wheat bread crumbs

1 pound ground turkey breast

¼ cup chopped fresh flat-leaf parsley

2 tablespoons chopped fresh tarragon, or ½ teaspoon dried

1 large egg, beaten

Glaze

2 tablespoons ketchup

1 tablespoon balsamic vinegar

2 teaspoons maple syrup

Preheat the oven to 400°F.

Heat the oil in a large skillet over medium-high heat. Add the onion and carrots and sauté until soft and onion is translucent but not browned, about 6 minutes. Add the garlic and cook until fragrant, about 1 minute longer.

Remove the vegetables from the heat and transfer to a large bowl. Add the lentils, ketchup, Worcestershire sauce, salt, and pepper and stir together. Add the bread crumbs, turkey, parsley, tarragon, and egg to the veggie mixture and lightly mix with your hands until all the ingredients are combined. Do not overwork. Transfer the mixture to a 9 x 5-inch loaf pan.

For the glaze, combine the ketchup, vinegar, and maple syrup and spread the glaze evenly over the top of the meat loaf. Bake until a meat thermometer reads 165°F, about 45 minutes. Remove from the oven and let rest for at least 10 minutes before cutting and serving.

To freeze uncooked: Freeze the loaf in the loaf pan (to hold shape) then remove, wrap tightly with plastic wrap, place the meat loaf back in the loaf pan and freeze for up to 3 months. To cook, bake the meat loaf until a thermometer reads 165°F, about twice the regular cooking time (approximately 90 to 100 minutes).

To freeze cooked: Let the loaf cool completely. Remove the loaf from the pan, then wrap the entire loaf tightly in plastic wrap or slice into individual pieces and wrap each. Then place entire loaf or slices in a large freezer bag. Defrost in the refrigerator or in the microwave, then reheat in the oven or microwave until hot.

Per serving: 272 calories, 21 g protein, 27 g carbohydrates, 4 g fiber, 9 g total sugar, 9 g fat, 2 g saturated fat, 505 mg sodium, 519 mg potassium (11% DV), 79 mg calcium (8% DV), 45 mg magnesium (11% DV), 1.03 mcg B12 (43% DV), 0.45 mg B6 (35% DV), iron 3.3 mg (12.2% DV)

# Zucchini Fritters

These fritters are a perfect snack to help meet your veggie servings for the day when you just don't have the time or energy to cook. Pop one or two out of the freezer, microwave for 30 to 60 seconds, and you've got a delicious veggie side or snack.

makes 6 servings (1 fritter each) / prep time: 15 minutes / total time: 25 minutes

**2 medium zucchini**

**½ teaspoon kosher salt**

**⅓ cup whole wheat flour**

**2 large eggs, beaten**

**½ cup sliced scallions**

**2 tablespoons grated Parmesan cheese**

**½ teaspoon garlic powder**

**⅛ teaspoon cayenne pepper (optional)**

**1 tablespoon olive oil**

Grate the zucchini into a medium bowl, using a food processor or a box grater. Sprinkle salt on the zucchini, gently toss to coat, and let sit for 10 minutes. Drain the zucchini completely by placing it on a clean dish towel or piece of cheesecloth and squeezing the water out. Return the zucchini to the bowl and combine with the flour, eggs, scallions, Parmesan, garlic powder, and cayenne. Mix with your hands until all the ingredients are well incorporated. Form the mixture into 6 patties.

Heat the oil in a large skillet over medium-high heat for 1 to 2 minutes. Working in batches of 3 or 4 at a time depending on the size of your skillet, cook the fritters until nicely browned and crispy, 3 to 4 minutes on each side, pressing down with a spatula after flipping once.

Let the fritters cool to room temperature, then freeze in a large freezer bag or in a container with wax paper between each layer.

Per serving (1 fritter): 90 calories, 5 g protein, 8 g carbohydrates, 2 g fiber, 1.5 g total sugar, 5 g fat, 1 g saturated fat, 150 mg sodium, 243 mg potassium (7% DV), 45 mg calcium (5% DV), 25 mg magnesium (6% DV), 0.253 mcg B12 (4% DV), 0.199 mg B6 (10% DV), 0.2 mg iron (1% DV)

# Minestrone Veggie Soup

This tomato-based classic soup has extra veggies and is straight-up comforting to eat. You may eat a couple of servings before freezing—but definitely save some for later. You'll be happy you did!

makes 6 servings / prep time: 15 minutes / total time: 45 minutes

---

2 tablespoons olive oil

1 cup chopped yellow onion

2 medium carrots, chopped

1 yellow bell pepper, chopped

1 cup cut green beans (1-inch pieces)

3 medium garlic cloves, minced

1 teaspoon dried oregano

1 teaspoon dried basil

¾ teaspoon salt

½ teaspoon freshly ground black pepper

4 cups low-sodium chicken broth

1 bay leaf

1 (28-ounce) can diced tomatoes, with their juice

1 (14-ounce) can crushed tomatoes

1 (15-ounce) can Great Northern beans, rinsed and drained

1 tablespoon balsamic vinegar

3 cups cooked whole wheat elbow pasta

½ cup grated Parmesan cheese

Heat the oil in a large Dutch oven over medium heat. Add the onion, carrots, bell pepper, and green beans and sauté until they soften, about 10 minutes. Add the garlic, oregano, basil, salt, and black pepper and stir to distribute evenly. Add the chicken broth, bay leaf, diced tomatoes, and crushed tomatoes and bring to a boil. Add the beans and vinegar and reduce to a simmer for 20 minutes. Remove and discard the bay leaf. Add ½ cup of the pasta to each serving and top with the Parmesan if eating immediately.

For freezing: Do not add the pasta to the soup. Let the soup cool in the refrigerator for at least 30 minutes. Portion into freezer containers with the label and date. Store for up to 2 months.

For thawing: Remove the soup from the container and place the frozen soup in a wide pot. Heat over low-medium heat, stirring and breaking the frozen soup up occasionally until the soup is heated through. Or, heat in a microwave-safe dish on high, stirring often, until the soup is steaming, about 5 minutes. To serve, add ½ cup cooked whole wheat pasta to each serving and top with the Parmesan.

Per serving: 336 calories, 18 g protein, 49 g carbohydrates, 9 g fiber, 7 g total sugar, 9 g fat, 2.5 g saturated fat, 655 mg sodium, 942 mg potassium (27% DV), 199 mg calcium (20% DV), 83 mg magnesium (21% DV), 0.351 mcg B12 (6% DV), 0.307 mg B6 (15% DV), 4.2 mg iron (23% DV)

# Hearty Vegetable Lasagna

The ultimate freezer-ready comfort food, this lasagna is not only delicious, but uses cottage cheese and ricotta cheese to add a meat-free boost of protein, so you'll feel satisfied long after eating it. Freezing in individual portions allows you to use what you need, when you need it, rather than having to thaw the entire lasagna at once.

makes 8 servings / prep time: 20 minutes / total time: 1 hour + 30 minutes cooling time

Cooking spray or oil

1½ tablespoons olive oil, divided

8 ounces cremini mushrooms, thinly sliced (about 2 cups)

1 cup diced onion

4 garlic cloves, minced, divided

1 teaspoon kosher salt, divided

1 cup diced carrots

1 medium zucchini, diced

1 (14.5-ounce) can no-salt tomato sauce

1 (14.5-ounce) can diced tomatoes

2 tablespoons tomato paste

½ cup fresh basil, chopped divided

½ cup fresh flat-leaf parsley, chopped, divided

2 cups 2% fat cottage cheese

1 cup part-skim ricotta cheese

2 large eggs

¼ teaspoon freshly ground black pepper

12 ounces shredded part-skim mozzarella cheese (about 3 cups)

½ cup grated Parmesan cheese

1 (9-ounce) package whole wheat no-boil lasagna noodles (we like DeLallo brand), or regular lasagna noodles, just follow the package directions for pre-cooking.

Preheat the oven to 350°F. Spray a 13 x 9-inch baking dish with cooking spray, or rub lightly with oil.

Add 1 tablespoon of the oil to a high-sided skillet over medium-high heat. Add the mushrooms, onion, half the garlic, and ¼ teaspoon of the salt. Sauté until the veggies begin to sweat out their moisture, about 6 minutes. Remove from the skillet and set aside in a small bowl.

Add the remaining ½ tablespoon oil to the skillet, along with the carrots, zucchini, and the remaining garlic. Sauté until soft and brown along the edges, about 5 minutes. Return the mushroom mixture to the skillet, and add the tomato sauce, diced tomatoes, tomato paste, and ¼ teaspoon of the salt. Simmer on

Healthy, Happy Pregnancy Cookbook

low for 15 minutes. Turn off heat and stir in ¼ teaspoon of the salt, ¼ cup of the basil, and ¼ cup of the parsley.

Combine the cottage cheese, ricotta, eggs, the remaining ¼ cup basil, the remaining ¼ cup parsley, the remaining ¼ teaspoon salt, and the pepper in a medium bowl.

Assemble the lasagna by coating the baking dish with a small amount of the veggie sauce. Add a layer of five lasagna noodles, overlapping the long edges to fit. Spread on another layer of the sauce, then a layer of the ricotta mixture, a thin layer of mozzarella cheese, and another layer of noodles. Repeat the process with three layers of noodles (sauce, ricotta, mozzarella, noodles.) Finish the top layer of noodles with the sauce, mozzarella, and Parmesan.

Bake the lasagna on the middle rack, loosely covered with foil, for 20 minutes. Remove the foil and bake, uncovered, until the middle is bubbling and the edges are browned, an additional 20 minutes. To lightly brown the cheese on the top, broil on high for the last 2 minutes of the cooking time.

Let the lasagna cool on the counter for 30 minutes, then refrigerate, covered, for at least an hour or overnight. Cut into even pieces and wrap each in plastic wrap. Then place the pieces together in a large freezer bag. Label with the name and date. Store for up to 2 months.

To reheat from frozen, remove the plastic wrap and microwave each piece until heated through, 4 to 5 minutes, or place in a baking dish and reheat at 350°F until heated through, 15 to 20 minutes.

Per serving: 400 calories, 27 g protein, 41 g carbohydrates, 3 g fiber, 10 g total sugar, 15 g fat, 7 g saturated fat, 668 mg sodium, 700 mg potassium (15% DV), 469 mg calcium (47% DV), 41 mg magnesium (10% DV), .8 mcg B12 (35% DV), .254 mg B6 (20% DV), 3.0 mg iron (16% DV)

# Mediterranean Lean Beef and Veggie Burgers

These burgers are inspired by flavors of the Mediterranean. They call for lean beef and include veggies as part of the patty, which means you get a burger that has major flavor and delivers veggies along with the protein. The burgers freeze well and thaw easily, making them great to have around post-baby.

makes 4 servings / prep time: 10 minutes / total time: 25 minutes

1 pound 90% lean ground beef

1 teaspoon minced fresh garlic

¾ cup finely chopped spinach

⅓ cup crumbled feta cheese

¼ cup chopped fresh flat-leaf parsley

½ teaspoon dried oregano

½ teaspoon dried rosemary

¼ teaspoon kosher salt

Add all the ingredients to a medium bowl. Mix with your hands just until combined, being careful not to overwork. Form the mixture into four ½-inch-thick patties.

Cut four squares of wax or parchment paper just slightly larger than the size of the burger; you want some overlap so it's easier to pull them apart after they're frozen. Stack the burgers with a sheet of paper between each one, then wrap tightly in plastic wrap. Place in a zip-top freezer bag with the name and date. Store in freezer for up to 3 months.

Before cooking, thaw in the refrigerator for 4 to 6 hours, or in the microwave on defrost just until thawed. Grill until the meat is cooked to an internal temperature of 145°F, approximately 5 minutes on each side. Serve on a whole grain roll.

Suggested toppings include red onion, tomato, lettuce, Greek olives, and 2% plain Greek yogurt.

Per serving: 237 calories, 25 g protein, 1 g carbohydrates, <1 g fiber, <1 g total sugar, 14 g fat, 6.5 g saturated fat, 291 mg sodium, 431 mg potassium, 93 mg calcium (19% DV), 33 mg magnesium (19% DV), 2.7 mcg B12 (45% DV), 0.5 mg B6 (32% DV), 5 mg iron (27% DV)

# Blueberry, Coconut, and Banana Cream Pops

It's nice to have a dessert waiting for you in the freezer, too! These creamy, "coconuty" pops will make your taste buds smile, and fill your belly, while baby is napping.

makes 6 pops / prep time: 5 minutes / total time: 5 minutes + overnight

1¼ cups frozen blueberries, thawed

1 cup canned unsweetened full-fat coconut milk

¾ cup unsweetened vanilla almond milk

2 bananas, cut into chunks

Blend the blueberries, coconut milk, almond milk, and bananas in a blender until smooth. Pour into 6 freezer pop molds and freeze overnight.

Per serving: 123 calories, 1 g protein, 13 g carbohydrates, 2 g fiber, 7 g total sugar, 9 g fat, 7 g saturated fat, 28 mg sodium, 236 mg potassium (7% DV), 48 mg calcium (5% DV), 27 mg magnesium (7% DV), 0 mcg B12 (0% DV), 0.135 mg B6 (7% DV), .5 mg iron (% DV)

CHAPTER NINE

# I'm Officially a Walking Snack Machine: Milk-Maker Meals

Making food for a tiny human using nothing but your body is pretty amazing. Because your body is working overtime (in more ways than one!), you're using major energy and probably feel like you want to eat everything in sight. The key is to fuel yourself with foods that provide protein and fiber—two very satisfying nutrients that can help sustain your blood sugar as you cater to the every whim of a tiny person. In addition, certain foods are considered galactagogues, or substances that promote lactation. You'll notice oats, chickpeas, nuts, and seeds used in these recipes, as they're thought to increase milk supply for some women. They're also really satisfying, which is a definite win-win for a nursing mom.

# Supermom Green Smoothie

     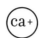

Kale and cucumber grace this smoothie with just a hint of "green flavor" while pineapple and apple add the perfect sweet balance. This smoothie packs in 1½ servings of veggies, 2 servings of fruit, protein, and omega-3 fats . . . all essential to keeping you energized, full of milk, and healthy while you take care of your little one.

makes 1 serving / prep time: 5 minutes / total time: 7 minutes

**1 cup coarsely chopped kale leaves**

**1 cup unsweetened almond milk, coconut milk, or 1% milk**

**1¼ cups frozen pineapple**

**½ cup cucumber**

**½ apple, chopped**

**1 tablespoon chia or hemp seeds**

**1 tablespoon unsalted natural almond butter or peanut butter**

**½ cup ice cubes**

Blend the kale and milk in a blender until combined. Add the pineapple, cucumber, apple, chia seeds, almond butter, and ice and blend until smooth, adding additional ice if necessary.

Per serving: 374 calories, 11 g protein, 47 g carbohydrates, 13 g fiber, 28 g total sugar, 18 g fat, 1.5 g saturated fat, 261 mg sodium, 816 mg potassium (17% DV), 711 mg calcium (71% DV), 130 mg magnesium (32% DV), 3 mcg B12 (125% DV), 0.5 mg B6 (36% DV), 4.3 mg iron (23% DV)

# Cocoa-Coconut Granola

Imagine a world where you can eat chocolate for breakfast and not get a sugar crash afterwards. This world exists. Meet your new favorite breakfast. While this breakfast packs in deep chocolate flavor, it also manages to deliver satisfying fiber and minimal added sugar. So you really can have your chocolate breakfast and eat it, too. Pair it with plain Greek yogurt or milk (cow or soy) to add protein for a complete meal. Or just nosh a serving as a snack, as is.

makes 4 servings (1 ¾ cups total) / prep time: 5 minutes / total time: 40 minutes

**Cooking spray or oil**

**1 cup old-fashioned rolled oats**

**1 tablespoon unsweetened cocoa powder**

**¼ teaspoon ground cinnamon**

**2 tablespoons maple syrup**

**1 tablespoon coconut oil**

**½ teaspoon pure vanilla extract**

**¼ cup cacao nibs**

**2 tablespoons unsweetened shredded coconut**

Preheat the oven to 275°F. Coat a baking sheet with cooking spray, or rub lightly with oil.

In a medium bowl, stir together the oats, cocoa powder, and cinnamon.

In a small bowl, whisk together the maple syrup, oil, and vanilla. Pour the liquid ingredients over the oat mixture and stir until fully coated.

Spread the mixture out in a single layer on the baking sheet and bake until it begins to get crispy, about 30 minutes.

Remove from the oven and stir in the cacao nibs and coconut. Spread out again in a single layer and bake until crisp all the way through, about another 10 minutes. Allow to cool fully before serving.

Per serving: 194 calories, 4 g protein, 25 g carbohydrates, 6 g fiber, 6 g total sugar, 10 g fat, 7 g saturated fat, 3 mg sodium, 127 mg potassium (4% DV), 26 mg calcium (3% DV), 38 mg magnesium (10% DV), 0 mcg B12 (0% DV), 0.029 mg B6 (1% DV), 1.6 mg iron (9% DV)

# Power Banana-Blueberry Pancakes

Traditional pancakes are delicious, but they are carb heavy, lacking the protein needed to keep you satisfied and energetic throughout the morning. Cottage cheese gives these pancakes added protein to balance out the carbohydrate and provide nice, steady energy all morning long.

makes 2 servings / prep time: 10 minutes / total time: 20 minutes

**1 banana**

**½ cup low-fat cottage cheese**

**2 large eggs**

**¼ cup 1% milk or unsweetened dairy-free alternative**

**½ teaspoon pure vanilla extract**

**½ teaspoon ground cinnamon**

**¼ teaspoon ground nutmeg**

**½ cup whole wheat flour**

**½ teaspoon baking powder**

**1 tablespoon coconut oil**

In a medium bowl, mash the banana and cottage cheese well with a fork. Whisk in the eggs, milk, vanilla, cinnamon, and nutmeg. In a separate bowl stir together the flour and baking powder. Add the wet ingredients to the flour mixture and stir to just combine.

Heat the oil in a medium skillet over medium heat. Pour the batter onto skillet, forming pancakes about 4 inches in diameter. Cook the pancakes for 3 to 4 minutes on each side. You'll know it's time to flip the pancakes when you see bubbles form on the surface.

Per serving: 380 calories, 22 g protein, 44 g carbohydrates, 5 g fiber, 15 g total sugar, 14 g fat, 8.5 g saturated fat, 356 mg sodium, 750 mg potassium (16% DV), 176 mg calcium (18% DV), 81 mg magnesium (20% DV), 0.242 mcg B12 (39% DV), 0.509 mg B6 (20% DV), 3.7 mg iron (20% DV)

# Date-Nut Breakfast Bars

If you want a nutritious, healthy, delicious breakfast—but you have zero time in the morning—make these bars ahead. They're 100% whole grain, loaded with fiber, and provide a boost of protein, to keep energy levels up and hunger levels down. And unlike most store-bought breakfast bars, these aren't loaded with sugar. In fact, the only sugar in these guys is from fruit!

makes 8 bars / prep time: 10 minutes / total time: 40 minutes

Cooking spray or oil

2½ cups old-fashioned rolled oats, divided

2 tablespoons ground cinnamon

⅛ teaspoon sea salt

2 teaspoons baking powder

3 large eggs

¾ cup unsweetened applesauce

½ cup unsalted natural almond butter

⅓ cup sunflower seed oil

½ cup coarsely chopped walnuts

½ cup finely chopped dates

Preheat the oven to 350°F. Coat a 9 x 9-inch baking dish with cooking spray, or rub lightly with oil.

Blend ½ cup of the oats in a blender or food processor until ground down to flour, about 1 minute.

In a large bowl, stir the oat flour, the remaining 2 cups oats, the cinnamon, salt, and baking powder together to combine.

In a separate bowl, stir the eggs, applesauce, almond butter, and sunflower seed oil until smooth.

Stir the egg mixture into the flour mixture until combined. Then gently stir in the walnuts and dates.

Pour the oat mixture into the baking dish and smooth the top. Bake until firm with a golden top, about 30 minutes. Allow to cool for 10 minutes before slicing into 8 equal, rectangular pieces.

Per serving: 389 calories, 10 g protein, 33 g carbohydrates, 7 g fiber, 9 g total sugar, 26 g fat, 3 g saturated fat, 169 mg sodium, 353 mg potassium (10% DV), 176 mg calcium (18% DV), 99 mg magnesium (25% DV), 0.242 mcg B12 (4% DV), 0.133 mg B6 (7% DV), 2.6 mg iron (15% DV)

# Creamy Quinoa-Flaxseed Cereal with Strawberries and Coconut

    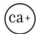

Oats are awesome, but they're not the only whole grain that makes a killer breakfast cereal. Quinoa is a complete protein, and cooking it up with milk adds even more protein to breakfast while the berries and coconut provide major flavor.

makes 4 servings / prep time: 5 minutes / total time: 35 minutes

1 cup uncooked quinoa

3½ cups 1% milk or soy milk

1 teaspoon pure vanilla extract

Dash of ground cinnamon

1 tablespoon honey

¼ cup ground flaxseed

1 cup sliced strawberries

¼ cup unsweetened shredded coconut

In a medium saucepan, combine the quinoa and 1½ cups of the milk and bring to a boil. Reduce the heat, cover, and simmer until the quinoa is tender, about 12 minutes.

Stir in the remaining 2 cups milk, the vanilla, cinnamon, and honey and return to a simmer. Simmer, stirring constantly, until the milk is mostly absorbed and cereal is thick and creamy, about 15 minutes more. Turn off the heat, stir in the flaxseeds, and leave the pan on the burner, covered, for 5 minutes.

Top the cereal with strawberries and coconut.

Per serving: 315 calories, 14 g protein, 47 g carbohydrates, 5 g fiber, 18 g total sugar, 9 g fat, 4.5 g saturated fat, 99 mg sodium, 665 mg potassium (19% DV), 300 mg calcium (30% DV), 124 mg magnesium (31% DV), 1.003 mcg B12 (17% DV), 0.329 mg B6 (16% DV), 2.5 mg iron (14% DV)

# Hemp Pita Pizzas with Mushrooms and Peppers

   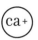 

In the time it would take to pick up the phone and order a pizza, these crispy personal pizzas will be out of the oven. And they taste really, really good. After trying these, you will likely be a believer in hemp seeds on savory foods. Serve each with a side salad or side of steamed veggies drizzled with olive oil for a full meal.

makes 2 individual pizzas / prep time: 5 minutes / total time: 5 minutes

**2 (6-inch) whole grain pitas**

**¼ cup marinara sauce**

**½ cup thinly sliced red bell peppers**

**½ cup thinly sliced mushrooms**

**½ cup shredded mozzarella cheese or dairy-free alternative**

**2 tablespoons hemp seeds**

Preheat the broiler to high.

Spread each pita with 2 tablespoons of the marinara sauce and top with ¼ cup of the peppers, ¼ cup of the mushrooms, and ¼ cup of mozzarella.

Broil until the cheese has melted and the pita is lightly browned, about 3 minutes. Sprinkle each pita with 1 tablespoon of hemp seeds.

Per serving: 406 calories, 20 g protein, 55 g carbohydrates, 9 g fiber, 5 g total sugar, 13 g fat, 4.5 g saturated fat, 731 mg sodium, 374 mg potassium (11% DV), 235 mg calcium (24% DV), 137 mg magnesium (34% DV), 0.66 mcg B12 (11% DV), 0.44 mg B6 (22% DV), 4.3 mg iron (24% DV)

# Salmon, Avocado, and Hearts of Palm Spinach Salad

If a salad is going to be a meal, it's got to have substance. No spindly salad is going to sustain a breast-feeding mama. Am I right? This salad provides two things most salads lack: protein and high-fiber carbs. And the protein comes from salmon, which delivers omega-3 fats that provide you with heart-healthy benefits and baby with brain-boosting benefits.

makes 4 servings / prep time: 5 minutes / total time: 5 minutes

3 cups baby spinach

3 (5-ounce) cans wild salmon, drained well and flaked

1 cup sliced hearts of palm (¼-inch disks)

2 cups corn kernels (fresh or frozen and thawed)

1½ ripe avocados, chopped

½ cup dried cranberries

3 tablespoons red wine vinegar

1 teaspoon Dijon mustard

½ teaspoon dried rosemary

¼ teaspoon coarse sea salt

¼ teaspoon garlic powder

Pinch of freshly ground black pepper

3 tablespoons olive oil

Place the spinach in a large salad bowl and top with the salmon, hearts of palm, corn, avocado, and cranberries.

Whisk together the vinegar, mustard, rosemary, salt, garlic powder, pepper, and oil.

Drizzle the dressing over the salad in the bowl and toss lightly to coat.

Per serving: 426 calories, 23 g protein, 35 g carbohydrates, 8 g fiber, 9 g total sugar, 24 g fat, 4 g saturated fat, 700 mg sodium, 892 mg potassium (25% DV), 239 mg calcium (24% DV), 91 mg magnesium (23% DV), 3.9 mcg B12 (65% DV), 0.564 mg B6 (28% DV), 3.3 mg iron (18% DV)

# B, L, T, A, H
# (Bacon, Lettuce, Tomato, Avocado, Hummus)

If you think a BLT can't get any better, prepare to be pleasantly surprised—mainly because avocado and hummus make EVERYTHING better. Because this lunch takes 5 minutes to prepare, you might even have spare time to catch a catnap, or finally wash your hair. And because this sandwich packs in major amounts of fiber, it will keep you satisfied long after you've cleaned your plate.

makes 2 sandwiches / prep time: 5 minutes / total time: 5 minutes

---

**Cooking spray**

**4 slices whole grain bread**

**½ avocado, mashed**

**4 tomato slices**

**2 slices center-cut bacon, cooked**

**2 large leaves romaine lettuce**

**2 tablespoons hummus**

Coat a large skillet with cooking spray and toast the bread in the skillet over medium-high heat until it's golden, about 2 minutes per side.

Spread two slices of the toast each with 1 tablespoon hummus and two slices of the toast each with ½ of the avocado. Cut the bacon slices in half and put two halves, side by side, on each slice of avocado toast, followed by 1 leaf of lettuce and 2 slices of tomato. Top the slices of toast with hummus.

Per serving: 410 calories, 6 g protein, 49 g carbohydrates, 12 g fiber, 8 g total sugar, 21 g fat, 6 g saturated fat, 438 mg sodium, 410 mg potassium (12% DV), 106 mg calcium (11% DV), 26 mg magnesium (7% DV), 0.14 mcg B12 (2% DV), 0.274 mg B6 (14% DV), 3 mg iron (17% DV)

# Broiled Soy-Ginger Flank Steak

Flank steak, a lean cut of beef, is marinated in a soy-ginger marinade and then broiled, mimicking the high direct heat that you would achieve with a grill. But there's no grill required! Serve it with our Seasoned Carrot Fries (page 119) and a side of roasted potatoes.

makes 4 servings / prep time: 15 minutes / total time: 25 minutes + 1 hour (or longer) marinating time

1¼ pounds flank steak or skirt steak

¼ cup reduced-sodium soy sauce

2-inch piece fresh ginger, peeled and grated

3 garlic cloves, chopped

1 teaspoon sesame oil

1 teaspoon Worcestershire sauce

½ teaspoon crushed red pepper flakes

½ teaspoon freshly ground black pepper

¼ teaspoon sea salt

Cut the steak into two even pieces. Combine the soy sauce, ginger, garlic, oil, Worcestershire sauce, red pepper flakes, black pepper, and salt in a large zip-top bag or a baking dish. Place the steak in the marinade and marinate, refrigerated, for at least 1 hour and up to 24 hours.

When ready to cook, remove the steak from the marinade. Turn the broiler on high and broil the meat on a broiler pan until it reaches an internal temperature of 145°F, 4 to 5 minutes on each side. Remove from the pan and transfer to a cutting board. Let rest for 5 minutes. Cut the steak, against the grain, into thin slices.

*Note:* This steak can also be grilled over medium-high flame for 4 to 5 minutes on each side.

Per serving: 281 calories, 30 g protein, 2 g carbohydrates, 0 g fiber, 0 g total sugar, 17 g fat, 6.5 g saturated fat, 500 mg sodium, 408 mg potassium (9% DV), 14 mg calcium (1.4% DV), 33 mg magnesium (8% DV), 3.27 mcg B12 (136% DV), 0.636 mg B6 (49% DV), 2.74 mg iron (10% DV)

# Slow Cooker Pork Loin and Vegetable Marinara over Whole Wheat Pasta

A classic Italian-style marinara with shredded pork, green pepper, and onions comes together fuss-free for a nutritious and easy weeknight dinner that you can prep and forget. This lean cut of pork becomes fall-off-the-bone tender (even though there's no bone) by way of this low-and-slow cooking method. Serve with a green salad, and dinner is ready.

makes 4 servings / prep time: 10 minutes / total time: 3 hours 10 minutes (or 7 hours 10 minutes for slow-cooking method)

1 pound pork sirloin tip roast

1 tablespoon olive oil

1 medium yellow onion, chopped

1 green bell pepper, chopped

2 teaspoons minced garlic

1 teaspoon dried basil

1 teaspoon dried oregano

1 (28-ounce) can fire-roasted diced tomatoes

1½ cups marinara sauce (see recipe on page 127, or store-bought such as Rao's)

½ cup white wine

½ teaspoon sea salt

¼ teaspoon red pepper flakes

4 cups (8 ounces) cooked whole wheat spaghetti

¼ cup freshly grated Parmesan cheese (optional)

Place the pork roast in a medium to large slow cooker. In a large skillet, heat the oil over medium-high heat. Add the onion and bell pepper and sauté until soft and the onion is lightly browned, about 10 minutes. Stir in the garlic, basil, and oregano, mix to combine, and cook another 2 minutes.

Add the cooked onion and pepper, the diced tomatoes, marinara, white wine, salt, and red pepper flakes to the slow cooker and stir everything to combine. Cook on low for 7 hours, or on high for 3 hours. Set the timer for 6 hours, or 2 hours, then 1 hour before it's done, take the pork out and cut into pieces and shred some of it. It might feel tough, but it will become tender in the next hour. Shred the rest of the pork roast with 2 forks in the slow cooker—it should shred easily.

Serve the pork with the sauce, spooned over cooked whole grain spaghetti. Top with Parmesan.

Per serving: 505 calories, 46 g protein, 62 g carbohydrates, 13 g fiber, 15 g total sugar, 8 g fat, 2.5 g saturated fat, 573 mg sodium, 408 mg potassium (26% DV), 70 mg calcium (7% DV), 88 mg magnesium (22% DV), 1.06 mcg B12 (44% DV), 0.901 mg B6 (69% DV), 3.5 mg iron (20% DV)

# Whole Roasted Chicken with Vegetables

This protein-rich, one-pan meal requires minimal prep work but yields results that will seem like you cooked all day. The leftover chicken can be used in stir-fries, salads, and fajitas. And a major bonus is that the leftover carcass can be used for homemade chicken stock, simply by boiling it with salt, any veggies that are on their way out, and a splash of vinegar.

makes 6 servings / prep time: 15 minutes / total time: 1 hour 10 minutes

1 (4- to 5-pound) whole roasting chicken

3 teaspoons olive oil, divided

1½ teaspoons sea salt, divided

½ teaspoon freshly ground black pepper

3 teaspoons dried herbes de Provence, divided

5 sprigs fresh thyme

1 lemon, sliced

5 garlic cloves

1 pound Yukon Gold potatoes, halved or quartered depending on size

4 medium carrots, cut into 1-inch pieces

1 large yellow onion, sliced into 1-inch chunks

Preheat the oven to 425°F. Remove the giblets from the cavity of the chicken. Pat the outside of the chicken with a paper towel to remove excess moisture. Brush the chicken with 2 teaspoons of the oil and sprinkle 1 teaspoon of the salt and the pepper. Rub 2 teaspoons of the herbes de Provence over the entire chicken. Stuff the cavity with the thyme, lemon slices, garlic, the remaining ½ teaspoon salt, and the remaining 1 teaspoon herbes de Provence. Truss the chicken by tying the ends of the legs together with kitchen twine so they rest gently over the breasts. Tuck the wing tips under so that they're not sticking out on the sides.

Add the potatoes, carrots, and onion to a roasting pan or a 9 x 13 baking dish. Drizzle the remaining 1 teaspoon oil over the vegetables and toss to coat. Place the chicken, breast side up, over the vegetables.

Cook for 55 to 60 minutes, or until the internal temperature reaches 165°F. Toss the vegetables once or twice throughout the cooking time. Let the chicken rest for 10 minutes before slicing.

Per serving: 427 calories, 39 g protein, 21 g carbohydrates, 4 g fiber, 4 g total sugar, 21 g fat, 5.5 g saturated fat, 430 mg sodium, 800 mg potassium (23% DV), 57 mg calcium (6% DV), 58 mg magnesium (14% DV), 1.28 mcg B12 (21% DV), .8 mg B6 (40% DV), 3 mg iron (17% DV)

Healthy, Happy Pregnancy Cookbook

# Garlic Shrimp, Balsamic Greens, and Tomatoes over Polenta

Store-bought polenta adds a fun, but easy, carb to this meal. The fresh veggies lend textures and flavors that are light yet satisfying. All the flavors meld into a perfectly balanced meal that provides a steady energy boost thanks to lean protein from the shrimp, carbs from the polenta, and a fiber boost from the veggies.

makes 3 servings / prep time: 5 minutes / total time: 20 minutes

---

1½ tablespoons olive oil

2 cups halved grape tomatoes

4 teaspoons chopped garlic

¾ teaspoon red pepper flakes

1 pound uncooked frozen shrimp, thawed, peeled, and deveined

6 cups arugula

¼ cup balsamic vinegar

½ teaspoon sea salt, divided

½ teaspoon freshly ground black pepper

1 tablespoon unsalted butter

1 tube store-bought polenta, cut into ¼-inch-thick slices

⅓ cup grated Parmesan cheese

Heat the oil in a large skillet over medium heat. Add the tomatoes, garlic, and red pepper flakes and sauté for 2 minutes. Add the shrimp, spacing it evenly in the pan, and cook until the shrimp turns opaque, about 1 minute per side.

Stir in the arugula and vinegar. Reduce the heat to low. Cook, stirring intermittently, until the arugula wilts. Season with ¼ teaspoon of the salt and the black pepper. Remove from the heat.

Heat the butter in a separate skillet over medium heat. Add the polenta slices and sauté until browned on both sides, about 2 minutes per side. Sprinkle with the remaining ¼ teaspoon salt. Serve the shrimp and arugula over the polenta, and top with Parmesan.

Per serving: 438 calories, 40 g protein, 36 g carbohydrates, 3.5 g fiber, 8 g total sugar, 15 g fat, 5.5 g saturated fat, 886 mg sodium, 835 mg potassium (18% DV), 306 mg calcium (31% DV), 90 mg magnesium (23% DV), 0.257 mcg B12 (11% DV), 0.16 mg B6 (12% DV), 3.5 mg iron (20% DV)

# Roasted Lemony Asparagus

Imagine asparagus drizzled with hollandaise sauce. Now imagine a much easier version that captures the same flavors but requires no sauce skills whatsoever. This dish is deceptively easy for as much flavor as it provides and makes a rockin' side dish for anything you throw its way.

makes 4 servings / prep time: 5 minutes / total time: 20 minutes

**1 large bunch asparagus (about 1 pound)**

**2 tablespoons olive oil, divided**

**2 teaspoons freshly squeezed lemon juice**

**½ teaspoon finely grated lemon zest**

**½ teaspoon coarse mustard**

**¼ teaspoon coarse sea salt**

**Pinch of freshly ground black pepper**

Preheat the oven to 400°F.

Toss the asparagus with 1½ tablespoons of the oil and lay out on a baking dish.

Roast until tender and just starting to brown, about 15 minutes.

Whisk together the remaining ½ tablespoon oil, the lemon juice, lemon zest, mustard, salt, and pepper.

Remove the asparagus from the oven, pour the lemon mixture on top, and toss lightly to coat.

Per serving: 83 calories, 3 g protein, 5 g carbohydrates, 2 g fiber, 2 g total sugar, 10 g fat, 1 g saturated fat, 80 mg sodium, 233 mg potassium (7% DV), 28 mg calcium (3% DV), 16 mg magnesium (4% DV), 0 mcg B12 (0% DV), 0.105 mg B6 (5% DV), 2.5 mg iron (14% DV)

# Herb-Roasted Root Veggies

Root veggies are high in carbohydrates, but also carry along antioxidants, vitamins, minerals, and fiber, making them a stellar carb choice. This dish is a great one to make on a weekend and then eat up throughout the week, and can be easily doubled. Plus, while the baking time seems long, the actual amount of time you need to be hands-on with this dish is minimal.

makes 4 servings / prep time: 5 minutes / total time: 1 hour 5 minutes

2 parsnips, cut into 1-inch pieces

2 carrots, cut into 1-inch pieces

1 rutabaga, peeled and cut into 1-inch pieces

1 medium onion, cut into quarters

2 beets, peeled and cut into 1-inch pieces

2 tablespoons olive oil

½ teaspoon coarse sea salt

½ teaspoon garlic powder

½ teaspoon dried oregano

½ teaspoon ground turmeric

½ teaspoon dried basil

¼ teaspoon freshly ground black pepper

Preheat the oven to 425°F.

Toss the parsnips, carrots, rutabaga, onion, beets, oil, salt, garlic powder, oregano, turmeric, basil, and pepper in a large baking dish. Roast until tender and golden, about 1 hour, stirring every 10 minutes.

Per serving: 170 calories, 3 g protein, 26 g carbohydrates, 7 g fiber, 13 g total sugar, 7 g fat, 1 g saturated fat, 262 mg sodium, 775 mg potassium (22% DV), 87 mg calcium (9% DV), 52 mg magnesium (13% DV), 0 mcg B12 (0% DV), 0.244 mg B6 (12% DV), 1.3 mg iron (7% DV)

# Flourless Chocolate Cake . . . with a Surprise!

A chocolate cake that uses no flour, boasts protein and fiber, AND actually tastes like a normal chocolate cake? Sign yourself up, lady. And, as if this cake needed more to brag about, it also freezes really well. Cut it into individual portions, wrap each in plastic wrap, and freeze for those days when you want a piece of chocolate cake but don't want to heat up the oven.

makes 8 servings / prep time: 10 minutes / total time: 40 minutes

**Cooking spray or oil**

**5 ounces bittersweet chocolate, chopped, divided**

**1 (15-ounce) can chickpeas, rinsed and drained**

**3 large eggs**

**1 teaspoon pure vanilla extract**

**½ cup sugar**

**¼ cup unsweetened cocoa powder**

**1 teaspoon baking powder**

Preheat the oven to 350°F. Coat a 9-inch round cake pan with cooking spray, or rub lightly with oil.

Reserve 1 ounce of the chocolate and heat the remaining 4 ounces in a double boiler, stirring until melted, about 7 minutes.

Puree the chickpeas, eggs, and vanilla in a blender or food processor until smooth, about 1 minute. Add the sugar, cocoa powder, baking powder, and melted chocolate and puree until all the ingredients are smooth, about 1 minute more. Stir in the reserved 1 ounce of chopped chocolate.

Pour the batter into the pan and bake until the center of the cake is just firm, 16 to 18 minutes. Do not overbake. Cool before cutting and serving.

Per serving: 229 calories, 6 g protein, 31 g carbohydrates, 6 g fiber, 19 g total sugar, 10 g fat, 5 g saturated fat, 157 mg sodium, 210 mg potassium (6% DV), 73 mg calcium (7% DV), 57 mg magnesium (14% DV), 0.274 mcg B12 (5% DV), 0.037 mg B6 (2% DV), 2.3 mg iron (13% DV)

Healthy, Happy Pregnancy Cookbook

# Oatmeal, Almond, and Cranberry Lactation Cookies

These cookies are not only delicious, they contain oats, brewer's yeast, and chia seeds, all foods that are reported to (anecdotally, not scientifically—many moms swear by these ingredients!) stimulate milk production. Whether it's something special in those ingredients, or simply that they're generally nutrient-rich, is not known, but either way these cookies offer a tasty way to make sure you're well nourished and able to produce plenty of milk for baby. Plus they're lower in sugar than a traditional cookie!

makes 30 cookies / prep time: 15 minutes / total time: 25 minutes

Cooking spray or oil

1 cup unsalted butter, softened, or ¾ cup warmed coconut oil

½ cup granulated sugar

½ cup packed brown sugar

2 large eggs

3 tablespoons molasses

1 teaspoon pure vanilla extract

1 cup whole wheat pastry flour

¾ cup almond flour or finely ground almonds

2 tablespoons brewer's yeast

1 teaspoon baking soda

1 teaspoon salt

1½ teaspoons ground cinnamon

3 cups old-fashioned rolled oats

½ cup dried cranberries

⅓ cup sliced almonds

3 tablespoons chia seeds

Preheat the oven to 375°F. Coat a cookie sheet with cooking spray, a light oil, or line with a nonstick silicone mat.

In a medium bowl, cream the butter, granulated sugar, and brown sugar. Beat in the eggs, one at a time, then stir in the molasses and vanilla.

In a separate bowl, combine both flours, the yeast, baking soda, salt, and cinnamon. Stir the dry ingredients into the creamed mixture. Mix in the oats, cranberries, almonds, and chia seeds.

Roll the dough into walnut-size balls, and place 2 inches apart on the cookie sheet.

Bake for 8 to 10 minutes. Allow the cookies to cool on the cookie sheet for 5 minutes before transferring to a wire rack to cool completely.

Per serving: 174 calories, 4 g protein, 19 g carbohydrates, 3 g fiber, 8 g total sugar, 10 g fat, 4 g saturated fat, 126 mg sodium, 100 mg potassium (6% DV), 33 mg calcium (3% DV), 32 mg magnesium (14% DV), .043 mcg B12 (5% DV), 0.08 mg B6 (2% DV), 0.9 mg iron (5% DV)

# Acknowledgments

Thanks to our recipe testers, particularly Dean Jarosh and Sharon Bookwalter and Diane Clarke (aka our moms!) whose love of food and knowledge in the kitchen not only helped us perfect these recipes, but whose guidance has shaped our love of food, family, and cooking.

A huge thank-you to Alison Fargis at Stonesong Literary Agency, who believed in this "little book that could" from the start. Her hard work, enthusiasm, and experience were instrumental in generating the interest in this book, and guiding us throughout the entire process of publishing it.

Thanks Julia Pastore and our editors at Atria Books, Donna Loffredo, Sarah Branham, and Leslie Meredith, and editorial assistant Haley Weaver, for their guidance and attention to detail. Thank you to all of the team at Atria for believing in the concept and helping us see it to fruition, especially Jackie Jou and Lisa Sciambra. Thanks also to Marjorie Korn for her keen editing skills.

From Stephanie: To my daughter, Juliette, who made me a mom, and guided me—pregnancy symptom by pregnancy symptom—throughout the process of creating this book so that I could relate to each recipe and topic on a personal level. To my mom and dad, who taught me how to love food and the importance of a good family meal. And to my husband, Jason, for (sometimes unknowingly) taste-testing many versions of these recipes, and unconditionally supporting me (and picking up extra daddy duty!) while I worked on this book with an infant in tow.

From Willow: To my dad, Dean Jarosh, our #1 hot cereal expert/recipe tester and always super-fan, Sharon (mom) whose grammar skills were invaluable, and Kalub, who sat through way too many versions of that breakfast cake. Jared, thanks for your patience, your taste buds, your genuine appreciation of food and eating, and for believing in me unfailingly. Todd, thanks for always being so sure this book would happen. Finally, thank you to all my clients who have let me tag along on their pregnancy adventures in our private practice.

Lastly, to each other, for working hard to make our first cookbook a reality.

# Index

# About the Authors

Stephanie Clarke and Willow Jarosh are nutrition experts, registered dietitians, and the co-owners of C&J Nutrition, a New York City– and Washington, DC–based nutrition communications company that provides nutrition counseling and consulting.

The pair are passionate about promoting wellness and happiness through daily food and lifestyle choices whether it's through counseling clients one-on-one, their company's national workplace wellness programs, or their work with the media writing articles, developing recipes, and appearing on national TV. The two are contributing editors at *SELF* magazine, a role they've held for six years, as well as healthy lifestyle experts for the Huffington Post.

Stephanie and Willow met in graduate school at the Tufts University School of Nutrition Science and Policy, where they both received masters degrees in nutrition communications and completed the dietetic internship program at the Tufts New England Medical Center.

After contributing recipes, meal plans, and nutrition content to numerous best-selling books, they're happy to present this as their first cookbook, for moms-to-be, new moms, and anyone who may know one!

Stephanie currently resides in Maryland, just outside Washington, DC, with her husband Jason, daughter Juliette, and white cat, Yogurt.

Willow lives in Manhattan with her boyfriend, Jared, and her hilarious calico cat, Luisa.